Prepared Childbirth
The Family Way

Throughout life we prepare for the things that really matter – school, career, marriage. Giving birth should be no exception. Because the birth event profoundly affects everyone involved, it deserves careful and thoughtful preparation. This manual was written to assist you in preparing for the birth of your child by reviewing material presented by your childbirth educator and offering guidelines for your own practice sessions. It reflects our philosophy that:

- childbirth is a joyful experience for which parents should prepare, and

- preparation should give a woman confidence in her body's ability to give birth.

As your knowledge increases, discussions about alternatives regarding labor and birth become more meaningful. Soon you will be able to make informed choices as you plan your approach to childbirth.

This is Prepared Childbirth – The Family Way

by

Debby Amis and **Jeanne Green**

For additional copies of this handbook, contact:

The Family Way Publications, Inc.

5804 Furneaux Drive
Plano, Texas 75093   USA

Phone: (972) 403-0297
Fax: (972) 403-1330
Web Site: http://www.thefamilyway.com
E-mail: info@thefamilyway.com

ISBN 0-9662875-7-6

Preface To The Sixth Edition

Prepared Childbirth – The Family Way was originally written in 1981 to provide a state-of-the-art handbook for the classes taught by The Family Way, Inc. Since that time we have continued to keep abreast of current childbirth research and trends so that educators and parents-to-be can continue to depend upon this manual to be current, concise, and complete. Six editions, along with annual updates, show our dedication to providing the best resource possible for educators and new parents. We welcome your comments and suggestions for this manual.

In Appreciation

If it were not for the volunteer efforts of Linda and Tom Arnold, who were attending our classes in 1981, *Prepared Childbirth – The Family Way* might never have been published. We will always be indebted to them for typesetting this book at a time when desktop publishing was the farthest thing from our minds. Their patience and untiring efforts in the many revisions made possible our first edition. Two other very special individuals, Jo Ann Moffitt, RN, and Vicki Mullen, PT, coauthors in our original publication, have our deepest thanks. Both of them have moved on to other endeavors in their respective fields, but we will always be appreciative of the energy and knowledge they shared with us in our early publications.

We would like to acknowledge the contributions of our talented artists: Vicki Wright drew the illustrations for the exercise sections, Stephen Brown prepared the outstanding anatomical illustrations, and Bob Mader, with our models Tina and Tomas Molander, provided the beautiful photographic images of comfort positions. Our lovely models on the birth balls are Margie Wallis, Nicole Allman, Tommie Black, Christy and Andrew McWhorter.

We are grateful to our husbands, who have truly made this a family-centered business. Steve Amis has been invaluable in designing the layout of our book so that revisions and updates can be easily accomplished. Gordon Green has shared his proofreading and editing skills as well as his medical expertise on care of the newborn.

For his contributions on epidural anesthesia, we thank Keith Reisler, M.D. For hours of consultation and review of the breastfeeding section, we thank Jeannette Crenshaw, IBCLC. The parents whose birth reports we feature contributed much to the spirit of this book. A special thank-you to all the wonderful childbirth educators we have worked with and learned from over the years – locally through The Family Way, and nationally through Lamaze International, the International Childbirth Education Association, and Doulas of North America. Lastly, we would like to thank the families in our childbirth classes who have shared their concerns, questions, tears, and joys of pregnancy and birth with us in The Family Way.

About The Authors

Debby Amis, a Fellow in the American College of Childbirth Educators, is certified as a childbirth educator by Lamaze International (formerly ASPO/Lamaze). She has taught childbirth education classes to families in North Texas for over twenty years. A longtime volunteer with Lamaze International, Debby is a past president of the Lamaze International Board of Directors and currently serves as Education Council Chair. Also certified as a doula, Debby has served as a labor support volunteer at Parkland Memorial Hospital and helped develop the curricula for the Lamaze International Labor Support Specialist Program, the Lamaze Labor Nurse Program, and the Childbirth Education for the 21st Century workshop. She is a faculty member for the Lamaze Childbirth Educator Program at the University of Texas School of Nursing at Austin as well as for Lamaze International. She has presented many workshops in childbirth education and labor support across the country.

Debby received her bachelor of science degree in nursing with highest honors from the University of Texas at Austin. At home, Debby has a husband, Steve; two sons, Brian and Ben; and one spoiled but lovable Springer Spaniel.

Jeanne Green began her career in childbirth education in 1975 as one of the first childbirth educators in the state of Arkansas. She helped to establish Prepared Childbirth, Inc. of Little Rock and became certified by ASPO/Lamaze (now Lamaze International). After moving to Texas in 1977, she founded and served as director and educator for The Family Way, Inc. Currently Jeanne serves on the faculty of both Lamaze International and the Lamaze International Labor Support Specialist Program. She is certified as a doula by Doulas of North America and is a Fellow in the American College of Childbirth Educators. She has presented workshops and sessions for numerous groups including Lamaze International and the International Childbirth Education Association.

When she is not teaching, writing, traveling, or attending births, Jeanne enjoys working in the laboratory for a pediatric practice. She holds a degree in biology from Trinity University and is registered as a medical technologist by the American Society of Clinical Pathologists. She and her husband Gordon have raised three daughters, Elaine, Whitney, and Emily, and a son, David. The empty nest has arrived – except for the bird!

Contents

Postpartum and Family

Birth Reports

Workbook

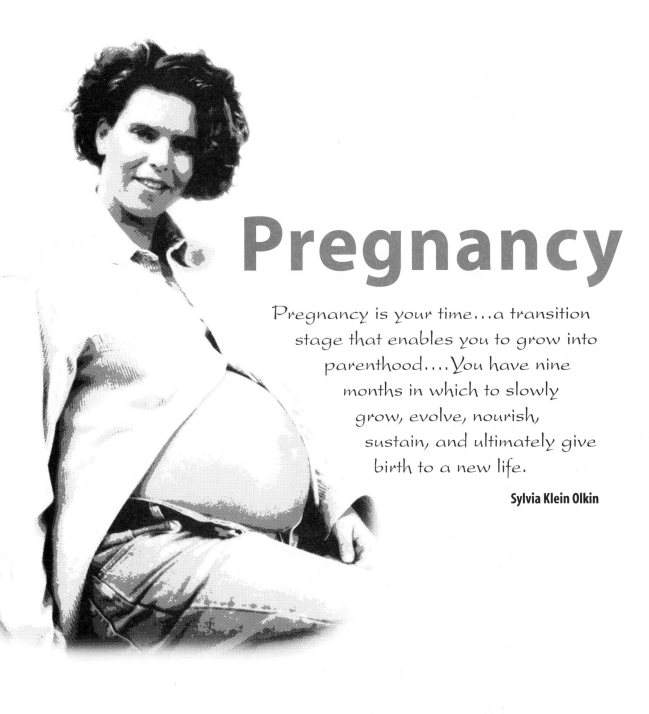

Pregnancy

Pregnancy is your time…a transition
stage that enables you to grow into
parenthood….You have nine
months in which to slowly
grow, evolve, nourish,
sustain, and ultimately give
birth to a new life.

Sylvia Klein Olkin

Communicate, Communicate, Communicate

Good communication is a key ingredient in a successful relationship. And listening is as important a communication skill as is speaking. Different personality types, different temperaments, and different sexes may communicate differently – and so may pregnant women!

For most, pregnancy is a time of good health, good feelings, heightened sexual pleasure, pride, and fulfillment. But intermixed with these good feelings are physical discomforts, emotional swings, worries about finances and added responsibilities, and perhaps a reluctance to leave behind a "carefree" life-style. Sometimes the father-to-be feels left out due to all the attention being focused on mom. Either or both partners may have negative feelings about mom's "new body." There are both increases and decreases in sexual desires during the course of pregnancy. If these changes of pregnancy are not discussed openly, misunderstandings, hostility, and guilt can be the result.

When two people are on the same wave length, thoughts or even words might escape your lips at the same moment. It is as though you are so connected that you hardly need to speak. At other times, you are so misunderstood you had just as well be speaking different languages.

It is the premise of John Gray in his book *Men Are from Mars, Women Are from Venus* that, "Not only do men and women communicate differently but they think, feel, perceive, react, respond, love, need, and appreciate differently. They almost seem to be from different planets, speaking different languages and needing different nourishment."

When a woman is pregnant she will learn a role in life that may be new to her – that of protector and nurturer for her growing baby. She may feel conflict between her need to relax and let go as her body changes, and her need to keep up her pace and image in the work-force. As she tries to do it all, her feminine needs are more exaggerated than ever. She needs to talk, to express her feelings, and to be reassured that she is competent and lovable. It may be difficult for her to ask for help. She may not understand her own mood swings, but she wants her partner to understand them. She needs him to be there for her – not to solve her problems as he is prone to do, but to listen to her as she unloads her joys and frustrations of pregnancy and her fears and anxieties of birth and parenthood.

She needs to understand that as much as she needs him to listen to her express her feelings, and for him to express his, he needs her to allow him to be silent. Women often think while they talk, but many men use silence and withdrawal to think. Don't mistake silence for rejection!

If you both try to understand one another's needs, you can continue to replace lost energy in each other's cup. If one person does all the giving, that cup will empty and the relationship will suffer. Riding the waves of the emotions of pregnancy and birth is not easy, but it can bring about a very special closeness and appreciation for one another and help establish a strong base for your new roles as parents.

Suggestions for the Pregnant Mother

- Some men prefer to focus on only one thing at a time. If you need to be listened to, or need help with something, he may appreciate it if you allow him to complete his current task before asking him to change his focus.
- Be direct when telling him what you need. He may be more than willing to help you, but he cannot be expected to read your mind, nor does he need lengthy explanations.
- Realize that most men need time alone with silence, with the TV, or the paper. Allow him this time to relax first, then he will more likely be patient when you need to be heard.
- It never hurts to compliment your partner and tell him how much you appreciate his help.

Suggestions for the Pregnant Father

- Listen to her stories of her day; ask for more detail even when you think there can be no more.
- Don't try to solve her problem unless she asks for a solution. Your physical presence, listening ears, and loving arms may be the only solution she needs.
- Reassure her; tell her you love her *and* her pregnant body.
- Support her; if you don't know what she needs, ask her.

What's Going On During Pregnancy

	Development of the Baby	Possible Feelings of the Mother	Possible Feelings of the Father
1st Trimester – Adjustment	**By the End of the First Month** Minus 14 days – last menstrual period Day 1 – fertilization Day 6 – implantation Day 14 – missed menstrual period ¼ to ½ inch long All organs present Day 18 – heart beating One month – arm and leg buds **By the End of the Second Month** Human facial features All major body systems laid down Particularly sensitive to chemicals Some doctors listen for fetal heart tones Capable of motion Arms, hands, fingers legs, feet, toes formed Real bone begins replacing cartilage Milk-tooth buds formed **By the End of the Third Month** Sex can be distinguished Less susceptible to outside forces Fetus kicking, making faces Fetus swallowing, breathing movements	**Physical** Hormonal upheaval Urinary frequency Fatigue Morning sickness Backache **Emotional** Excitement Apprehension Mood swings Cries for anger or joy	**Physical** "Couvade" – may experience physical symptoms similar to mom **Emotional** New sense of responsibility Concerned with mother's mood swings
		Both Mother and Father Pride Often ambivalence precedes acceptance of pregnancy Concerned over mother's changing body Sometimes ambivalent to sex	
2nd Trimester – Acceptance	**By the End of the Fourth Month** Fetus quite recognizable as a human baby Length: 8 to 10 inches Weight: 6 ounces **By the End of the Fifth Month** Quickening – mother feels movement Length: 10-12 inches Weight: about 1 pound Hair on head Lanugo (fine hair) covering body Nails on fingers and toes Fetal heart tones (FHT) clearly audible **By the End of the Sixth Month** Possible chance of survival if born now Length: 14 inches Weight: 1¾ pounds Vernix caseosa produced Permanent tooth buds formed Strong grip	**Physical** Hormones in better balance More energy Quickening – feels baby move **Emotional** Less moodiness Feelings of good health and well-being	**Physical** Hears heart tones Feels baby move **Emotional** Gets more emotionally involved Becomes more protective of mother
		Both Mother and Father Sex more appealing Fear of injury to baby Worry over partner	
3rd Trimester – Anticipation	**By the End of the Seventh Month** Weight: 3 pounds Gaining immunities from mother Shedding lanugo **By the End of the Eighth Month** Weight: 5 pounds Probably head down position Gaining immunities from mother **By the End of the Ninth Month** Length: 20 inches Weight: 7 to 7 ½ pounds Lightening – baby "drops" Gaining immunities from mother	**Physical** Discomforts due to enlarging body Fatigue May not have much interest in sex **Emotional** Body image – feels "glowing" and/or unattractive Nightmares	**Physical** Sees baby move **Emotional** May feel left out Financial worries Concerns over sexual relationship
		Both Mother and Father Excitement about impending birth mixed with fears for well being of mother and baby Apprehension about birth experience Concern about parenthood and loss of freedom	

Try This for Comfort

Discomfort	Solution
Nausea	Eat 4 or 5 small meals a day rather than 3 large meals. Don't let stomach become empty. Eat crackers before arising. Chew crystallized ginger; drink ginger tea. Wear motion sickness bands. Eat well balanced diet – especially B vitamins.
Fatigue	Listen to your body – Rest!
Stuffy nose	Try saline nose drops. Use warm compresses.
Backache	Maintain proper posture. Use good body mechanics. Try pelvic tilt exercises.
Constipation	Eat lots of foods with bulk – whole grains, bran, raw vegetables, fresh and dried fruits. Drink lots of water and fruit juices. Establish a daily habit. Get regular exercise such as walking.
Leg cramps	Partner can place the heel of mom's foot in his palm, then gently use his forearm to push the ball of her foot towards her body. Adjust calcium/phosphorus ratio – talk to doctor or midwife. Help prevent with calf stretches (page 15.)
Heartburn	Eat small frequent meals; drink more liquids between meals rather than with meals. Avoid fatty and highly spiced foods. Avoid lying down immediately after a meal. Avoid ice cold, very hot, or carbonated beverages. Talk to your doctor or midwife about using antacids.
Shortness of breath	Maintain correct posture. Slow down. Sleep propped up with pillows.
Swelling in legs and feet	Sit, swim, or walk in water. Increase fluids. Sit instead of stand; lie down instead of sit; elevate feet several times a day. Do foot twirls. Apply support hose after legs have been elevated.
Varicose veins	Elevate legs at right angle to body 2 to 5 minutes several times a day. Wear support hose. Try warm bath to soothe legs. Avoid "knees-locked" and legs crossed positions.
Hemorrhoids	Avoid constipation. Kegel for circulation. Apply witch hazel compresses.

Some Helpful Terms

Amniotic sac or "bag of waters." The thin membrane which encloses the baby and the amniotic fluid. At full term, there is roughly a quart of amniotic fluid surrounding the baby. About one third of this fluid is constantly being replenished every hour.

Braxton-Hicks contractions. Usually painless uterine contractions present from the earliest days of pregnancy which the mother may feel from about the fifth month on. These contractions help to enlarge the uterus. They may occur more frequently and become greater in intensity as the mother gets closer to the start of true labor.

Contractions. The rhythmic tightening and relaxation of the uterine muscles which results in the effacement and dilation of the cervix and the eventual expulsion of the baby. True labor contractions usually come in a regular pattern, gradually get closer together, and gradually increase in intensity. The frequency of the contractions is measured from the beginning of one contraction to the beginning of the next contraction; the duration refers to length of one contraction; and the intensity refers to the strength of the contraction.

Cervix. The lowest portion of the uterus which resembles a "neck" until birth, when it opens into the birth canal (or vagina) to allow passage of the baby.

Dilation (dilatation). The opening up of the cervix so that the baby can pass from the uterus to the vagina or birth canal. Measured in centimeters from 0 to 10.

Doula. A professional labor support person or postpartum helper. (See page 29.)

Effacement. The thinning and shortening of the cervix. In the primigravida, effacement is usually complete before the cervix begins to open up. Measured in percentages from 0 to 100.

Endorphins. The body's own morphine-like pain inhibitors which are produced in high levels during an un-medicated labor and birth.

Engagement. The entrance of the baby's presenting part into the upper oval of the mother's pelvis. In primigravidas, engagement often takes place about two weeks before the baby's birth. In multigravidas, it can occur as late as the onset of labor.

Episiotomy. A small surgical incision of the perineum made to enlarge the vaginal opening. If an episiotomy is necessary, it is done just before the birth of the baby.

Fundus. The top or uppermost portion of the uterus.

Lightening. The sensation the mother feels when the baby "drops" down or gradually settles into the pelvis as the presenting part becomes engaged.

Multigravida. A woman pregnant with her second or subsequent child.

Multipara (multip). A woman who has given birth to more than one child.

Perineum. The external tissues surrounding the urethra, vagina, and anus; the space between the vagina and anus. The elasticity of these tissues varies with the individual and has a bearing on whether or not an episiotomy needs to be done.

Presentation. Refers to the part of the baby which can first be felt through the cervix upon vaginal exam; the part of the baby which will first enter the birth canal:

- *Cephalic or vertex.* Head first – occurs in more than 95% of births. May be anterior, posterior or transverse position.

- *Breech.* One or both feet or buttocks first – occurs in 3.5% of births.

- *Shoulder (transverse lie).* Baby lying sideways in the uterus – occurs in less than 1.5% of births.

Primigravida. A woman pregnant with her first child.

Primipara (primip). A woman who has given birth to her first child.

Station. The relationship of the baby's presenting part to the mother's ischial spines (part of the pelvis). A minus 3 station refers to a baby whose presenting part has not yet entered the pelvis or is floating; a 0 (zero) station refers to a baby whose presenting part is engaged; and a plus 4 station refers to a baby whose presenting part is at the perineal floor and delivery is imminent.

Anatomy of Pregnancy

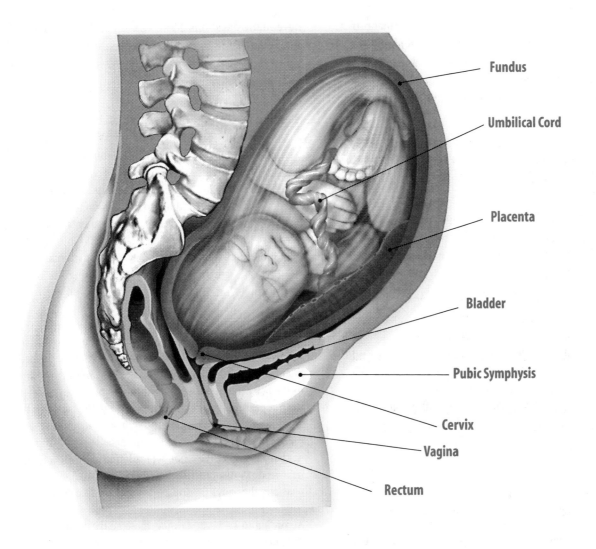

Fundus

Umbilical Cord

Placenta

Bladder

Pubic Symphysis

Cervix

Vagina

Rectum

Presentations

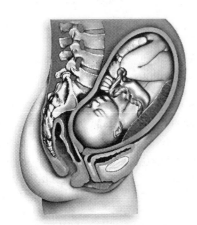

Anterior Position

The most common position
for the baby to be born

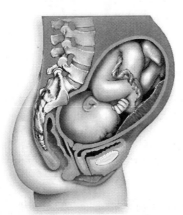

Posterior Position

"Sunnyside-up" – associated
with back labor

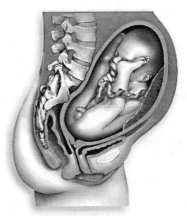

Frank Breech

Most common breech position

Precautions

Pregnancy and breastfeeding are healthy, normal processes for most women. However, during pregnancy and breastfeeding, the developing baby is vulnerable to potential toxins which may be transmitted to the baby through the mother. For this reason, pregnant and nursing women have many questions about what is and what may not be safe. Below are some guidelines for the substances asked about most commonly. Your health care provider can provide additional information.

	Pregnancy	Breastfeeding
Alcohol	Because safe levels for alcohol consumption have not been established for pregnant women, most health care providers recommend that pregnant women avoid alcoholic beverages altogether during pregnancy. Heavy consumption of alcohol, especially in the early months of pregnancy, is associated with fetal alcohol syndrome which may include mental retardation, facial malformations, growth retardation, and liver and kidney abnormalities.	According to the American Academy of Pediatrics, an occasional drink or regular light drinking (one or fewer drinks per day) have not been found to be harmful to the nursing baby. However, alcohol is passed freely into breastmilk and studies have shown that nursing mothers who abuse alcohol may have babies who fail to grow and develop normally.
Tobacco	Maternal smoking reduces the amount of oxygen delivered to the baby in utero, which may impair the growth of the baby. Maternal cigarette smoking has been linked to 20 to 30 percent of all low birth-weight babies in the United States. Low birth-weight is the second leading cause of infant deaths in this country.	According to La Leche League, for the mother who smokes twenty or fewer cigarettes per day, the benefits of breastfeeding outweigh the small health risks of transmitting nicotine to the baby in the breastmilk. However, the more cigarettes the mother smokes, the greater the risks to the baby. For the nursing mother who is unable to quit smoking, it is recommended that the mother smoke immediately after nursing her baby to reduce the amount of nicotine in her milk for the next feeding. Also, the mother should reduce (eliminate, if possible) the baby's passive exposure to tobacco smoke.
Caffeine	Although caffeine does cross the placenta to the baby, it does not appear to be linked with birth defects. According to a 2001 news release by the American College of Obstetricians and Gynecologists (ACOG), "there's no proof that small amounts of caffeine (for instance, 1 or 2 cups of coffee daily) cause problems during pregnancy." Most caffeine-containing teas and sodas contain about a third to a half as much caffeine as coffee.	According to La Leche League, the amount of caffeine in 5 (5 ounce) cups or less of coffee does not cause problems for most breastfeeding mothers and their babies. Greater amounts of caffeine may cause overstimulation of the baby.
Legal Drugs	Because the safety of prescription drugs as well as many over-the-counter medications may depend on the stage of pregnancy and/or other substances or medications the woman may be taking, pregnant and breastfeeding women should consult with their health care provider before taking any medication.	
Illegal Drugs	Illegal drugs including heroin, marijuana, and cocaine may have devastating effects on the developing baby in utero. Pregnant women are strongly urged to avoid all "street" drugs and to seek treatment if they have addictions.	According to the American Academy of Pediatrics, women who use heroin, marijuana, or cocaine should be discouraged from breastfeeding because of the potential dangerous effects of these drugs which are transmitted in breastmilk. However, women who are taking 20 mg. or less of methadone to combat heroin addiction can and should breastfeed their babies.

Nutrition

There is no more important issue in pregnancy, to both mother and baby, than nutrition. It has been said that the mother is "eating for two," and that is literally the case. The unborn infant's growth is dependent upon what mom takes into her body. If the maternal diet consists of good growth materials, baby will be the beneficiary. If the diet is inadequate, or if mom takes in harmful elements (drugs, alcohol), then the baby is the unsuspecting recipient. Attention to the mother's diet is among the most critical matters in your pregnancy.

Recommended Weight Gain

According to *Nutrition During Pregnancy* released by the National Academy of Sciences, the most important determinant of the recommended weight gain during pregnancy is the woman's pre-pregnancy weight-for-height. Women who are underweight before becoming pregnant are encouraged to gain 28 to 40 pounds during pregnancy; normal weight women are encouraged to gain 25 to 35 pounds; and overweight women are encouraged to gain 15 to 25 pounds. Your health care provider may have specific recommendations for you based on your medical history and life-style.

Recommended Daily Food Intake:

In addition to the recommended servings on the U. S. Department of Agriculture food guide pyramid, most researchers agree that a pregnant woman needs approximately 300 extra calories a day to provide for the growth of the baby and maternal changes. One extra serving from the *Milk, Yogurt, and Cheese* group and one extra serving from the *Meat, Poultry, Fish, Dry Beans, Eggs, and Nuts* group can easily provide these extra calories. Examples of healthy food choices from each group are included on the next two pages.

Precautions/Foods to Avoid

According to a 2001 ACOG news release, pregnant women should avoid unpasteurized milk or soft cheeses, and undercooked or raw meat, fish, shellfish, or eggs. (Sufficient heat kills bacteria and parasites that could cause harm to the developing baby.) All fresh fruits and vegetables should be washed thoroughly before eating. The FDA advises that pregnant and nursing women eat a variety of small fish rather than large fish such as shark, swordfish, and king mackerel. Larger fish are older, so may accumulate high levels of mercury. Fish contain many valuable nutrients, but intake should be limited to 12 ounces of cooked fish per week while pregnant or nursing.

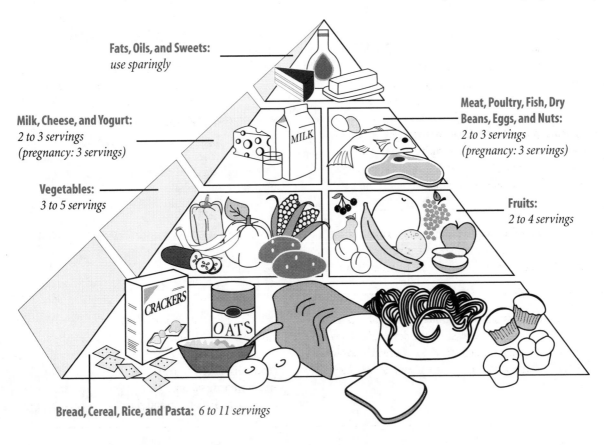

Fats, Oils, and Sweets: *use sparingly*

Milk, Cheese, and Yogurt: *2 to 3 servings (pregnancy: 3 servings)*

Vegetables: *3 to 5 servings*

Meat, Poultry, Fish, Dry Beans, Eggs, and Nuts: *2 to 3 servings (pregnancy: 3 servings)*

Fruits: *2 to 4 servings*

Bread, Cereal, Rice, and Pasta: *6 to 11 servings*

Healthy Food Choices

Bread, Cereal, Rice, and Pasta *6 to 11 servings daily*	Many of these choices are high in complex carbohydrates; vitamins such as B vitamins (including folate) and vitamin E; minerals; and fiber. Eat products from a variety of grains such as wheat, oats, rice, and corn. Choose whole-grain foods rather than processed or fortified foods. When reading labels, look for *whole-wheat* as the first ingredient for breads, crackers, pasta, and cereals, rather than *wheat flour*. Not all brown bread contains whole-wheat and not all whole-wheat crackers are brown. Look at the label rather than the color.
Vegetables *3 to 5 servings daily*	Vegetables provide carbohydrates; vitamins such as vitamin A, vitamin C, and folate; minerals such as iron and magnesium; and valuable fiber. They are naturally low in fat and calories. To insure that you meet your needs for the various vitamins, it is important to choose from a variety of vegetables. Eat deep yellow and dark green leafy vegetables often. To obtain the most vitamins, choose vegetables in this order: fresh, frozen, canned.
Fruits *2 to 4 servings daily*	Fruits also provide carbohydrates; vitamins such as vitamin A, vitamin C, and folate; minerals such as potassium; and valuable fiber. Although fruit juices are healthy beverages, you will get additional vitamins and fiber by eating the whole fruit. Choose citrus fruits, melons, and berries regularly to make sure you are getting enough vitamin C.
Milk, Yogurt, and Cheese *2 to 3 servings daily* *pregnancy: 3 servings* *breastfeeding: 3 servings*	Milk products provide protein, vitamins A and D, and minerals such as calcium and phosphorus. Serving sizes for dairy products are determined by calcium content. Because cottage cheese is lower in calcium than most other cheeses, one cup of cottage cheese counts as only ½ serving of milk. On the other hand, ricotta cheese is much higher in calcium so that only ½ cup counts as one serving of milk. If you have trouble digesting milk, you may need nutritional counseling to insure that you get all the nutrients you need from this food group.
Meat, Poultry, Fish, Dry Beans, Eggs, and Nuts *2 to 3 servings daily* *pregnancy: about 3 servings* *breastfeeding: about 3 servings*	For the pregnant woman, the number of servings from the protein group varies according to her choices. The Recommended Daily Allowance (RDA) for protein during pregnancy is 60 grams. Some protein choices are excellent sources of protein *(chicken breast, 3½ oz. = 29 grams; tuna, 3 oz. = 23 grams)* while other choices are poorer sources *(bacon, 2 slices = 4 grams; fast-food fish sandwich = 14 grams)*. Complete proteins are needed for growth and development of the baby. Animal sources (meat, milk, and eggs) provide complete proteins, while plant sources of protein (grains, dried beans, seeds, and nuts) are incomplete proteins. You must combine incomplete proteins from differing sources to make complete proteins. If you are a vegetarian, you may need nutritional counseling to make sure you are getting all the nutrients you need.
Fats, Oils, And Sweets *use sparingly*	We do need some fat in our diet in order to metabolize foods properly and absorb certain vitamins. However, it is easy to get too many fats and the wrong kinds of fats in our diet. For salad oils, spreads, and cooking oils use olive oil or canola oil as first choice, vegetable oils (corn, safflower, sunflower) as second choice. Least preferred are saturated fats such as palm and coconut oil and fats from animal sources. Because most processed sweets add only empty calories and/or fats to your diet, fruits are better choices for desserts and snacks.
Supplements	According to *Nutrition During Pregnancy,* released by the National Academy of Sciences, normal, healthy pregnant women should be able to obtain most needed nutrients from diet alone. The only supplements that healthy, pregnant women may need are low doses of iron and folic acid. The American College of Obstetricians and Gynecologists (ACOG) does NOT recommend restriction of salt during pregnancy.
Water	Pregnant women have up to 40% more blood volume by the time they reach term. To support this increase in blood volume, pregnant women need extra fluids. Milk, fruit juices, and water are the recommended beverages. ACOG recommends at least 8 glasses of water per day during pregnancy.

Sample Serving Size	Healthy Ideas
1 slice of bread, muffin, small roll ½ bagel or ½ English muffin One tortilla ½ cup cooked cereal, pasta, or rice 1 ounce processed cereal (read package) 4 to 8 crackers (depending on size, content) 3 cups of popcorn	100% whole-wheat products have more B vitamins and fiber than either brown or white wheat flour bread or crackers. Corn tortillas contain less fat and fewer calories than flour tortillas. Baked corn chips have much less fat than fried chips. Make pancakes or waffles from whole-grain flour or add wheat bran to the batter. Oatmeal and shredded wheat are two high nutrition cereals. Cheese melted on mini shredded wheat squares, air popped popcorn, and rye or whole-grain crackers make good snacks.
1 medium sized vegetable 1 cup raw leafy greens ½ cup cooked vegetables ½ cup of vegetable juice	Salsa and pico de gallo may be enjoyed with a meal or as a snack to add vitamins A and C. Leafy greens (the darker, the better) such as spinach, broccoli, Brussels sprouts, and lettuces are high in vitamins A and C and folate. Tomatoes and green and red peppers used in salads or sauces are good sources of vitamin C. Make your plate as colorful as possible and you will more easily get the nutrients you need.
1 medium-sized fruit ½ large fruit ¾ cup fruit juice ½ cup canned fruit	Fruits make excellent snacks and desserts. Choose fresh fruits; 100% fruit juices; and frozen, canned (in its own juice), or dried fruits. Avoid fruits canned in heavy syrup unless you are trying to add extra calories to your diet.
1 cup milk 1 cup yogurt ½ cup some soft cheeses such as ricotta 1½ ounces of hard cheese such as cheddar ½ cup ice cream, custard, or pudding	Calcium quantities are not affected by fat content, so whenever possible choose the nonfat or lowfat item for heart-healthy eating. Even most frozen desserts are available in lowfat or nonfat varieties. If you are trying to increase weight gain, try the harder cheeses and whole milk products.
3 ounces cooked lean meat, poultry, or fish 2–3 eggs 1-1½ cup cooked beans 4-6 tablespoons peanut butter ⅔-1 cup nuts 1 cup tofu (soybean curd)	*Complete proteins (animal sources).* For heart-healthy eating, chicken, turkey, fish, liver, lean pork, and lean beef are all good sources. Egg whites or egg substitutes may be used in cooking or baking, as well as for breakfast or in salads. *Incomplete proteins (plant sources).* Some popular ways to combine incomplete proteins to make complete proteins include: cereal with milk, macaroni with cheese, red beans with rice, split pea soup with whole-grain crackers, and peanut butter on whole-wheat bread.
1 tablespoon (1 pat) butter = 14 grams of fat 1 tablespoon mayonnaise = 12 grams of fat 1 cup of 2% milk = 5 grams of fat 1 cup of ½% milk = 1 gram of fat 1 ounce of hard cheese = 8 grams of fat 1 egg = 6 grams of fat 3 ounces skinless chicken = 4 grams of fat 3 ounces lean sirloin beef = 7 grams of fat	The recommended energy intake for the average pregnant woman is 2500 calories a day. The maximum recommended fat intake is 30% or 750 calories (approximately 83 grams of fat). To determine the number of calories from fat in a food, multiply the number of grams of fat by 9. To determine the percentage of calories from fat in a food, divide the number of calories from fat by the total number of calories in the food. Read food labels carefully and aim for no more than 30% of your daily calories from fat.

Do you know?...

. . . good nutrition in pregnancy is linked with

- *healthier babies*
- *more energy (less fatigue)*
- *better pattern of weight gain (and weight loss postpartum)*
- *less premature labor*
- *greater elasticity of tissues (less need for episiotomy)*
- *more rapid healing after birth.*

Body Mechanics

There are four main factors which accompany pregnancy that make body awareness and protection essential. The increased blood volume can contribute to muscle aches and swelling and/or decreased sensations in the legs and arms. Hormones being released to soften ligaments also add to muscle aches. The added weight of the baby pulling forward on the uterus where it attaches to the low back can cause increased back discomfort. These muscles need to be maintained and allowed to rest. The baby's presence also changes the mother's center of gravity. The following two pages of exercises and suggestions for daily activities should help decrease discomforts now, in labor, and throughout life for both men and women. The partner, as well as the pregnant woman, should perform these activities daily.

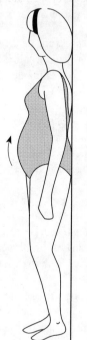

Standing Posture

Stand with feet about 3 inches apart with toes turned slightly outward.

Keep hips tucked under (pelvic tilt).

Keep shoulders back but do not let the back arch.

Keep head back over shoulders.

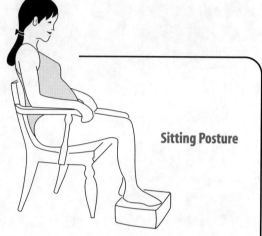

Sitting Posture

Sit in a chair with a firm but comfortable back support, with head over shoulders.

Arm rest should not be too low or too high.

Keep knees slightly higher than hips.

Small pads behind neck and low back may be added for comfort.

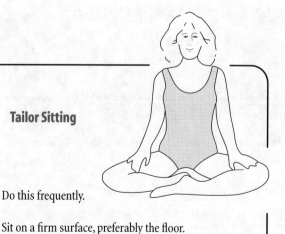

Tailor Sitting

Do this frequently.

Sit on a firm surface, preferably the floor.

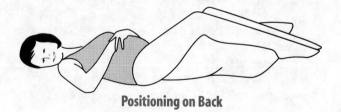

Positioning on Back

Place 2 or 3 pillows under knees.

Place a rolled bath towel under the bend of neck. If using a pillow at the head, also place it well under the shoulders.

Keep arms at sides or resting on stomach.

Lying on back recommended only prior to 20 weeks or during postpartum.

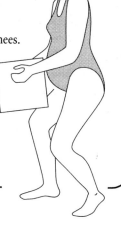

Stooping, Lifting, and Carrying Objects

Place one foot ahead of other before bending at knees.

Straighten legs, keep back straight.

Lift object slightly to one side.

Carry object waist high, close to body.

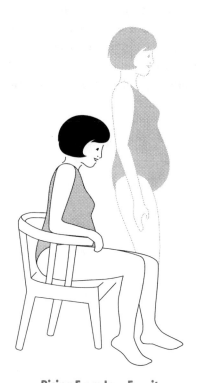

Rising From Low Furniture

Scoot hips forward to edge of chair.

Place one foot slightly forward and rotate hips in the
direction of forward foot.

Keep back straight.

Use arms and large thigh muscles to lift yourself up.

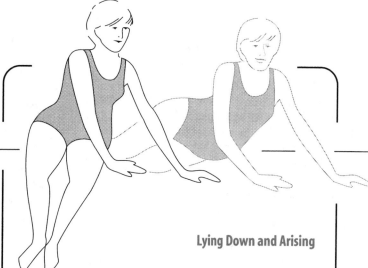

Lying Down and Arising

From sitting position, use hands to walk self down to
side-lying.

If rolling to back, turn shoulders and hips as one unit.

Return to side-lying again as one unit.

Pause for a moment before rising.

Side-Lying

Lie on side with knees bent.

Place pillow between knees, under upper arm, under head,
and under uterus as needed for comfort.

Lower arm may either be in front under pillow or behind
the back. ;

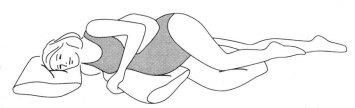

Birth Fitness Exercises

Perform all exercises slowly without bouncing or jerking. Stretching should not be done to the point of pain. Start with a small number of repetitions and gradually increase to your individual tolerance. It does not take long exercise sessions to ease aches, increase flexibility and circulation, and generally make you feel better. These exercises can be done while watching television or during short stretch breaks throughout the day (see page 88).

All pelvic tilt exercises may be done to ease backache during pregnancy and labor. The pelvic tilt on all fours may be helpful in rotating a posterior baby when done in the last month of pregnancy or during labor.

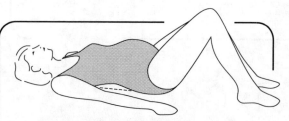

Pelvic Tilt on Back (prior to 20 weeks)

Lie on back with knees bent.

Tighten the stomach muscles pushing the low back flat against the floor.

Hold for 5 counts; relax; repeat.

Variation:
While holding the pelvic tilt, bring one knee towards the chest. Grasp the knee with both hands and pull towards the chest until you feel a good stretch (not pain) in the back muscles.

Hold 30 seconds, then return leg to starting position and repeat with other leg.

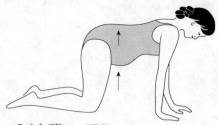

Pelvic Tilt on All Fours

Assume all fours position keeping back straight (do not let lower back sag).

Tighten the stomach muscles so pelvis tucks under and lower back rounds.

Hold for 5 counts; relax; repeat.

Variation:
Hold the pelvic tilt while you "swish" hips from side-to-side. Head turns as if ear will touch hips on the same side.

Repeat each side.

Standing Pelvic Tilt

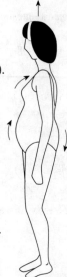

Stand with knees softened (slightly bent).

Tighten stomach and press the small of the back flat, as if against an imaginary wall.

Hold this position for one minute.

Relax.

Repeat often if standing for long periods.

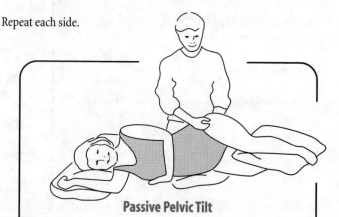

Passive Pelvic Tilt

Mom lies on her side with knees bent. Partner positions himself behind mom's hips.

Using his hand nearest her head, he places his palm on the crest of her hip.

His other hand is placed on her tail bone.

He slowly rotates the crest of her hip back toward himself.

Release – repeat.

Wall Stretch

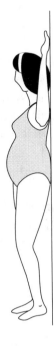

Stand against the wall with knees slightly bent.

Place shoulders, elbows, and wrists against the wall with elbows bent and fingers pointing upwards.

Slowly slide arms up the wall, straightening elbows.

Once arms are overhead, try to pull abdomen up and in so the back flattens against the wall.

Slide arms back down to the starting position.

Relax abdominals.

Repeat.

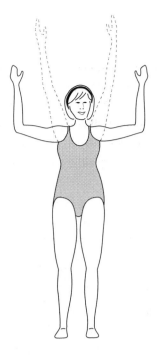

Calf Stretch Against Wall

Stand 2-3 feet back from wall.

Move left foot in towards wall. Pull in abdomen. Bend left knee, placing hands on wall. Lean in towards wall, keeping head, chest, hips, and right heel in a straight line.

Hold 30-60 seconds while feeling a mild stretch in the right calf.

Change legs and repeat.

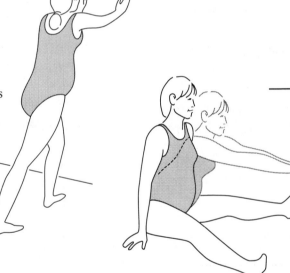

Tailor Stretch

Tilt pelvis and maintain it.

Extend legs with knees straight. Extend both arms and reach forward slowly until you feel a mild stretch.

Return to starting position.

Repeat.

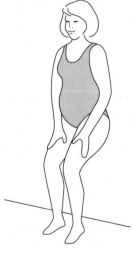

Wall Squat

Hold a standing pelvic tilt position with back against a wall.

Slowly slide upper body down the wall until knees are bent as if sitting on a stool.

Hold this position with contracted thighs and abdominals while relaxing all muscles not being used.

Add:
1. Tighten and release pelvic floor.
2. Use the contracted thighs to simulate uterine contractions while practicing breathing patterns.

Slowly return to standing position.

Kegel Exercises

Most people are completely unaware of the existence of the pelvic floor or pubococcygeus (PC) muscle until they attend prepared childbirth classes. The benefits of achieving and maintaining good tone in this muscle are many and include:

- Prevention of urinary "dribbling" when coughing or laughing.

- Possible prevention of need for surgery later in life to pull up a "sagging" uterus or other pelvic organs.

- Decreased discomfort from pelvic exams.

- A shortened and much easier second stage labor (actual birth of the baby).

- Improved healing of perineum from episiotomy repair and/or hemorrhoids.

- Greater pleasure during sexual intercourse.* Regular exercise every day can strengthen the PC muscle. This has enabled some women to reach orgasm more consistently during intercourse. These exercises done by men can help sustain erections to allow the woman more time to achieve orgasm.

- In men, a possible decrease in likelihood of developing prostate problems by enhancing circulation and support.

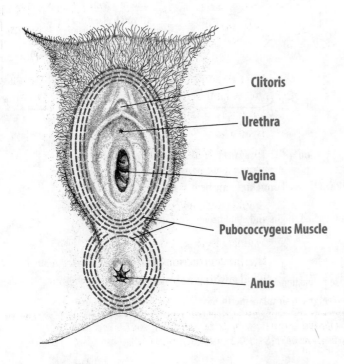

- Clitoris
- Urethra
- Vagina
- Pubococcygeus Muscle
- Anus

The pelvic floor muscle stretches from the pubic symphysis in front to the "tailbone" in back and forms a "sling" of support for the bladder, the uterus, the vagina, and part of the rectum. The muscle fibers are interlocking and surround the opening of the bladder (urethra), the vagina (vaginal orifice), and the rectum (anus).

To identify the correct muscle, sit on the toilet with legs spread apart. Begin to urinate, then contract the muscle necessary to stop the flow of urine; hold; release. Repeat until you learn to control the PC muscle. After you have determined that you are contracting the correct muscle, do not start and stop the flow of urine except as an occasional check. Practice the following exercises on a routine basis after emptying the bladder, or incorporate practicing into any daily routine such as answering the phone, driving a car, standing in line, etc.

To strengthen the PC muscle, these variations of the Kegel exercise are recommended:

Flicks – Contract, then release the PC muscle for one to two seconds (contract for one-two seconds; release for one-two seconds; repeat). Do these contractions in groups of ten; about ten times each day.

Extended Kegel – Contract the PC muscle and *hold*. Begin by contracting as tightly as you can for 5 seconds and work up to holding for 20 seconds. The muscle may tire after one extended Kegel, so do these at intervals throughout the day, up to ten times each day. Form a good life-long habit of tightening the PC muscle right after you urinate.

Elevator Exercise – Imagine that your pelvic floor muscle is an elevator. Contract the muscle and slowly increase the tension as you go up in the elevator – second, third, fourth, and finally to the fifth floor. Now, slowly release the tension in the pelvic floor muscle going down in the elevator – fourth, third, second, first floor, and basement. The basement is where the muscle should be at the actual moment of birth. Finally, contract back to the first floor level and maintain this tone at all times.

Physical therapists who specialize in women's health are good resources for pelvic floor problems as well as other discomforts of pregnancy.

---

* See *Woman's Experience of Sex* by Sheila Kitzinger

ACOG Guidelines for Exercise

Because of impressive recent research on the benefits of exercise, ACOG now recommends 30 minutes or more of moderate exercise on most, if not all, days of the week for pregnant women without medical complications. Participation in a wide range of recreational activities appears to be safe. Of course you should avoid activities with a high risk of falling or for abdominal trauma, such as skiing or contact sports. Spurts of heavy exercise followed by long periods of no activity put strain on your body and offer few benefits.

Research also shows that exercise may be beneficial in the prevention of gestational diabetes. Your goal should be to reach or keep a safe fitness level during pregnancy.

Start your workout routine with slow, low-impact activities such as walking or cycling. Wear the right shoes with good padding and support for your activities. Wear a sports bra that fits well and gives good support. Your breasts are growing and may be very tender. Drink plenty of fluid before, during, and after your workout.

Avoid jerky, bouncy, or high-impact motions. Jumping, jarring motions or quick direction changes can strain your joints and cause pain. Low-impact exercise such as walking or swimming is best.

Avoid deep knee bends, full sit-ups, double straight-leg lifts, and straight-leg toe touches which could strain the abdominal and back muscles.

Get up slowly after lying or sitting on the floor. Once you're standing, walk in place briefly. After 20 weeks of pregnancy, don't do any exercises on your back. Also avoid motionless standing, because your blood circulation could decrease and cut down the blood flow to your baby.

Be sure to take a break if you need one. If you have trouble talking normally during your workout, ease up. Never exercise until you are exhausted.

Follow intense exercise with cooling down for 5-10 minutes. Slow your pace little by little and end your workout by gently stretching. Don't stretch too far, though. This can injure the tissue that connects your joints.

Reduce your workout levels in late pregnancy. Exercise that may have been easy earlier in pregnancy becomes harder as your belly expands.

The type of exercise you can safely do depends on your health and fitness level. Pregnancy is not the time to take up a new sport. If you were active before getting pregnant, though, you should be able to keep it up, within reason. A return to physical activity after pregnancy has been associated with decreased incidence of postpartum depression.

Certain sports are safe even for beginners. Others are OK for those who have done them for a while. Still others are off-limits during pregnancy. With any type of exercise you'd like to try, be sure to discuss it with your doctor ahead of time. Here are some options:

- *Walking.* If you were not active before getting pregnant, walking is the ideal way to start an exercise program. Try to walk briskly for 30 minutes most , if not all, days of the week.
- *Swimming.* This is great for your body because it works many different muscles. The water supports your weight so you avoid injury and muscle strain. Stay off the diving board, though. Hitting the water with great force can be harmful
- *Jogging.* If you were a runner before you became pregnant, you can keep hitting the road now. Be careful, though. Avoid getting too hot. Stop if you feel tired or any pain. Drink plenty of water to replace the fluid you lose in sweat.
- *Aerobics.* Low-impact aerobics is a safe and good way to keep your heart and lungs strong. There are aerobics classes designed just for pregnant women. Water aerobics also is a good class to try. It combines the benefits of swimming and aerobics.

Signs of a Problem

If you have any of these symptoms when you exercise, stop your workout and call the doctor:

- Dizziness or faintness
- Headache
- Increased shortness of breath
- Irregular or rapid heartbeat
- Chest pain
- Trouble walking or calf pain, swelling
- Pain
- Vaginal bleeding
- Uterine contractions that continue after rest
- Fluid gushing or leaking from your vagina

Adapted from *ACOG Committee Opinion: Exercise During Pregnancy and the Postpartum Period* by the American College of Obstetricians and Gynecologists (ACOG): Washington, DC, © 2002 and *Planning Your Pregnancy and Birth* by ACOG: Washington, DC, © 2000.

On the Ball!

Benefits of using a "Birth Ball" before, during, and after labor

When you sit on a ball, the abdominal and lower back muscles are used to help you keep your balance. Your pelvis tilts forward, which encourages the baby to move into a good position. While sitting on the ball, moving your hips for comfort and balance comes naturally. Rocking the pelvis and shifting weight in the upright position can increase blood circulation, lessen back pain, and improve posture. The gentle pressure of the ball may help relieve discomfort from hemorrhoids and pressure on the pelvic floor. Rocking or gentle bouncing may comfort your baby before and after birth! Try sitting on a ball at a desk or while watching TV, as well as using one in an exercise program.

How to use a "Birth Ball" safely

While sitting on the ball, you should be barefooted or wearing rubber soled shoes. The ball should fit like a chair. Hips, knees, and ankles should each be bent to 90°. Because your center of gravity changes during pregnancy, you should have a source of support near you while using the ball, to provide balance if you need it.

Positions and Movements to Try

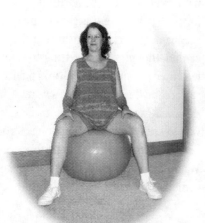

Begin moving in a circular or figure-eight motion while sitting on the ball. This relaxes the back and pelvic areas and helps you to establish your balance. Add pelvic tilts, moving forward and back, or side-to-side.

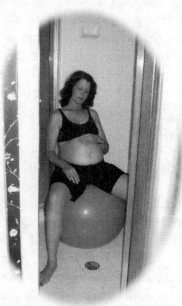

The ball may be taken into the shower to sit on while you enjoy the sensations of the warm water.

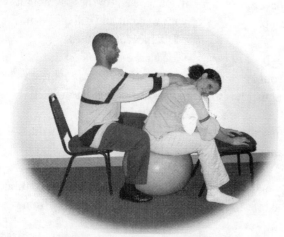

Sit on the ball and lean forward relaxing on a pillow placed on a table, bed, or chair. This helps relieve back pain by moving the baby forward.

Kneel on the floor or on the bed with the ball in front of you. Lean over the ball, rolling it forward and back to find a comfortable position for your upper body to rest. Your arms may hug the ball, or be relaxed hanging over it. Your partner may apply back pressure to help relieve pain.

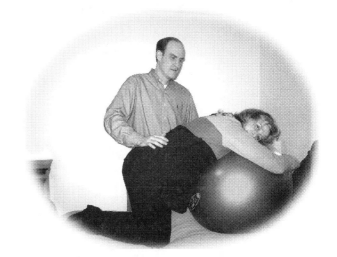

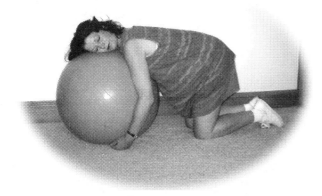

A kneeling position allows for free movement of the pelvis, while gravity encourages the largest and heaviest part of the baby to rotate off mom's back to an anterior position. Putting the weight of the upper body on the ball keeps weight off the wrists.

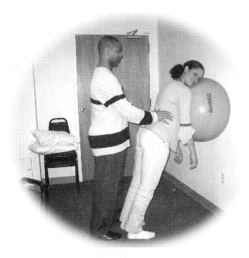

Standing while leaning on a ball that is placed on the wall, a bed, or table, encourages pelvic swaying and rotation, which may help relieve pain and encourage the baby to descend. Standing, with your back on the ball against the wall offers pleasant pressure for an aching back, or support for a wall-squat position.

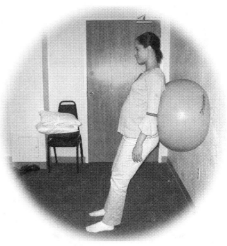

Sitting on the ball, lean back into your partner who is sitting on a chair behind you.

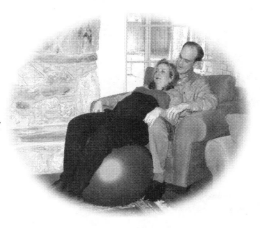

Comfort Positions for Pregnancy and Labor

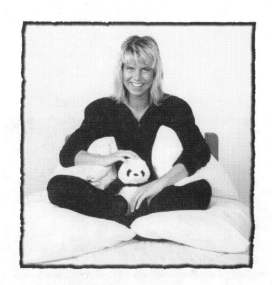

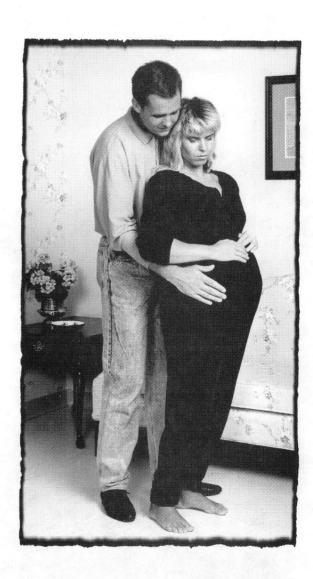

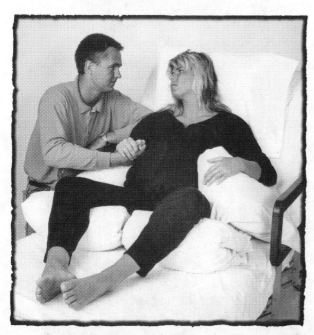

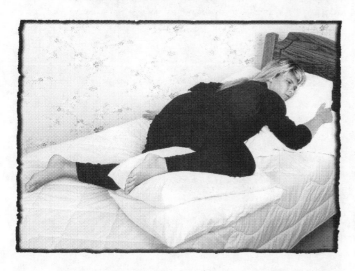

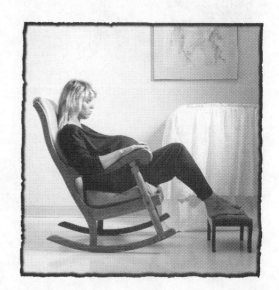

Comfort Positions for Pregnancy and Labor

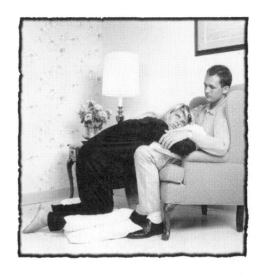

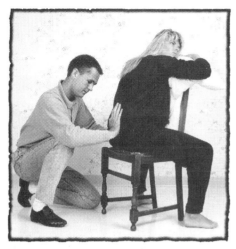

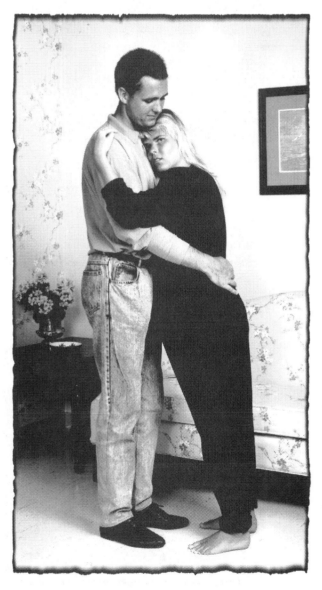

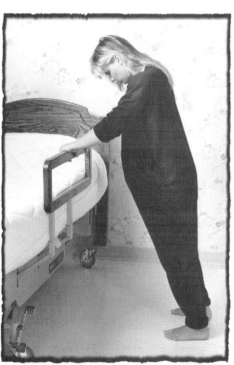

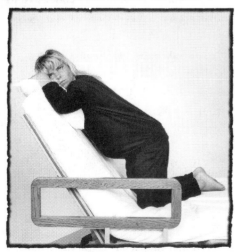

Active Relaxation Techniques

Active relaxation is an important foundation upon which many of the comfort techniques in prepared childbirth are built. This is not the ability to "tune out" and fall asleep, but the ability to "tune in" to one's body and to control the release or relaxation of muscles. This does not come easily to all people, but with practice anyone can consciously relax. Different people respond to different relaxation techniques. You will be taught several methods in your classes. Practice each technique, and after you have mastered them, use what works best for you. Relaxation is not an exercise for labor and delivery only, but also for the weeks, months, and years following birth. When any stressful situation arises (dentist visits, freeway driving, baby crying, medical procedures, etc.) think *relax*; you will gain control over your body and reduce stress and/or pain. Become conscious of your state of relaxation at all times (see page 87).

Partner's Role

The best way for the partner to help someone else relax is for him to be able to relax himself. Make practice time a team effort; both of you learn to relax and both learn to check for areas of tension. Talk about what increases relaxation and what provokes tension in each of you. You may learn some interesting things about one another. The tone of your voice and the firmness of your touch can affect relaxation in your mate. The partner should look for tension, feel for tension, and coax tension away with both verbal cues and touch.

Setting the Stage

While it is both possible and desirable to be able to relax in either chaos or calm, it is easier to learn the techniques when the environment is conducive to it. When first preparing for a practice session (and also when you are in labor), think of calming all your senses. Check the following and adjust for maximum comfort:

- sight – lighting dim or comfortable
- sounds – music or silence
- smell – fragrances or fresh air
- taste – water, flavored ice, mouthwash
- touch – temperature (fan, heater)
- touch – texture (blanket, pillow)

Get Ready to Relax

- Environment check
- Quick body scan
- Tension release exercises
- Comfortable position
- Focus
- Deep, relaxing, cleansing breath

After you have adjusted your environment, scan your body from head to toe. If you find a tense or painful spot, attempt to release tension with exercises like head rotations (left, forward, right), shoulder rolls, shaking arms and hands, ankle rolls, and pelvic tilts.

Find a comfortable position with every part of your body supported and joints bent. Use pillows under head, knees, and arms. Practice relaxing in sitting, side-lying, and semi-reclining positions. As your ability to relax improves, practice in walking and standing positions also. You will labor in all these positions .

Signal your body to relax by selecting a focal point and taking a cleansing breath. Use the various techniques of progressive relaxation, selective relaxation, touch relaxation, autogenic phrases, and visual imagery. Suggested practice sessions may be found in the workbook section on pages 92-94.

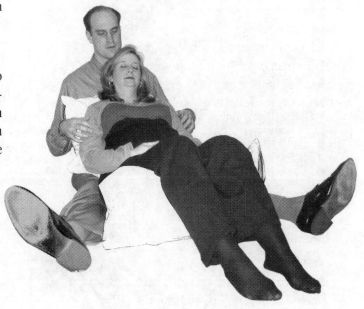

Progressive Relaxation

Progressive relaxation, as its name implies, is the technique of progressing through the body releasing one muscle group at a time until the entire body is consciously relaxed. At first it may be helpful to locate tension in muscles by either contracting or stretching them to feel their presence (see *Progressive Tense/Release* practice exercise on page 92). Master this practice exercise so that you reach the point where you can simply release by mentally progressing down your body as in the following scenario.

- Begin by relaxing the muscles of your head and face. Release down the back of your neck, across your shoulders and arms, down your chest, abdomen and back, all the way down your legs to your toes. Breathe slowly, releasing more and more with each exhalation. Each time you release a muscle, concentrate on the positioning of that muscle and on the feeling of complete relaxation.
- It may help to think of a comforting touch smoothing gently from your brow, up into your hair, over the top of your head, and down your body.

Selective Relaxation
Neuromuscular control

Selective relaxation consists of contracting one muscle group while keeping all other muscles relaxed. When the uterus contracts during labor, there is a tendency for the other muscles of the body to contract in response to it. Tension travels through the body, sapping energy and increasing pain. Selective relaxation serves as a rehearsal for labor. The muscle you hold tight simulates a uterine contraction as you learn to relax all other muscles. It takes practice to learn this skill, but the benefits will show in labor. It is most helpful for the partner to check for relaxation. Example:

Contract right arm … *release* all other muscles
 …*release* right arm

Contract jaws … *relax* the rest of the body
 … *release* jaws

Contract abdominals and pelvic floor … *release* pelvic floor … *release* abdominals

Contract left arm, right leg … *release* other muscles … *release* right leg, left arm

Autogenic Phrases

The repetition of descriptive phrases can induce relaxation as you concentrate on each part of your body. Analyze how relaxation feels to you, then describe those sensations. You may use the same sensation for each muscle group:

- my feet are warm,
- my hands are warm,
- my shoulders are warm;

or describe each muscle with a different sensation:

- my hands feel warm,
- my arms are loose,
- my feet are heavy.

You may say the phrases aloud or silently, or you may listen to someone read them. Pause between phrases. Use phrases that are positive for you so that you refresh yourself with this exercise. For some pregnant women, the *last* thing they want to feel is warm and heavy! You may add some positive affirmations about your baby and your general state of well-being when you do this exercise. My baby is strong and healthy…. I feel peaceful and calm (see *Relaxing Words* on page 93).

Visual Imagery

Visual imagery is a journey of the mind to a relaxing place. Its purpose is to reduce tension by concentrating on a mood and a place apart from your present situation, rather than focusing on your muscles as in other relaxation techniques. Create images that to you are peaceful and calming, and will therefore reduce muscular tension and lead to relaxation. You could imagine yourself in any relaxing place, real or imaginary: a warm, sandy beach; on a bearskin rug in front of a fireplace; or floating on clouds. Bring into your image sights, sounds, textures, tastes, colors, and scents that are relaxing to you. To be most effective during labor, you and your partner should thoroughly acquaint yourselves with your images or journey so that key words or phrases can help you return to a relaxed state (see *Relaxing Images*, page 94). You are totally in control. Be creative.

Touch Relaxation

Touch relaxation is one of the most important tools a labor partner will use during actual labor. With pressure, kneading, rhythmic stroking, or counterpressure, he can help mom release tense muscles. Practicing these techniques now will condition mom to release to touch during labor and will teach the partner how to touch, stroke, massage, and press in the most effective ways. Some women enjoy and relax well to touch throughout labor and others don't wish to be touched at all during certain periods. Communicate your needs and use your own adaptations of these techniques during practice and actual labor.

Gentle Pressure

As contractions increase in intensity, you may notice tightening of the brow, eyes, jaw, or hands. Gentle pressure, with or without movement, can help her identify and release that tension.

For overall tension – give her a strong bear hug and let her release into you.

Kneading

Slow rhythmic kneading is helpful for reducing tension in the shoulders, thighs, or buttocks. Grasp the muscle between the heel of your hand and your closed fingers. Squeeze in with gentle pressure, hold, then release and repeat, moving across the muscle. The thumbs may be used with the heel of the hand, but avoid pinching with thumb and fingers.

Stroking

Hand over hand stroking is effective on the back, thighs, or lower abdomen. Use firm pressure with the palm of the hand to stroke from shoulder to hip, or thigh to knee. Before one hand leaves the body, the other hand begins a second stroke. Alternate hands, maintaining constant contact with mom as you slowly move across her back or thigh. Hand over hand across the lower abdomen may be done by mom during a contraction – it is a natural response to rub where it hurts.

Encircling the arm with two hands at her shoulder, squeeze gently, moving down the arm to the tips of the fingers with one long continuous stroke. Use the same technique from upper thigh to the toes. She will release her tension to your touch if her limbs are fully supported or her arms are hanging by her side. Do not drop her arm or leg as you release the fingers or toes.

Counterpressure

This sustained, generally heavy pressure, is effective on painful areas of the lower back. Fold your fingers flat against the palm of your hand. Keeping wrist straight, use the knuckles of that fist to press against her pain. Position yourself so your body will lean into your arm to increase the pressure from your fist. The heel of the hand may be used for counter pressure, but it is more uncomfortable on the wrist for long periods.

Sample Exercise

Frown … release as partner strokes across forehead with fingers, or lays palm across it

Clench teeth … release to pressure of palms cupping jaw or to stroking of jaw

Tighten arm … release one muscle group at a time – biceps, forearm, hand, and fingers as partner strokes with two hands encircling arm

Clench fist … release fingers as partner opens fingers and squeezes or massages hand

Hunch shoulders … release to kneading or downward pressure of hands on shoulders in rhythm to exhalations

Arch back … release to steady pressure or massage

Pull in abdominal muscles … release to hand-over-hand stroking on lower abdomen

Tighten legs … release to long stroking of the thighs, calves, and feet

Putting It All Together
Total Body Release With Practice Contractions

After you have learned all these relaxation techniques, you should be able to release your whole body on command. Progress from being able to relax in the ideal environment to letting go of tension while standing at the kitchen sink or sitting at a desk . Try as you may, you will not have a distraction-free environment during labor! When the partner says "contraction begins," he is giving a verbal cue for mom to relax and breathe. The partner should be alert for possible signs of tension and use the tools of verbal cues ("Relax your jaw"), visual imagery ("Remember the warmth of the beach"), and touch to encourage relaxation. A pain stimulus such as holding a hand in ice water can be used to simulate a contraction. As you continue to practice and master the various relaxation techniques, you will notice improvement in your ability to cope with "practice contractions."

Womb Mates

Giving birth to multiples – twins, triplets, or more – is certain to multiply the joy to parents in the long term. However, along with added joy comes added risk and added precaution. When two or more babies share a womb, it expands to accommodate them – and so must mom. It is amazing what a body can do. But as you might expect, many of the challenges of pregnancy are exaggerated along with the increase in size and number of babies.

Proper body mechanics and exercises for posture are particularly important when the center of gravity is so changed by a large abdomen. With added weight, more stress is put on the back. Sturdy flat heeled shoes and a maternity girdle may help to ease discomforts. Pelvic tilts on hands and knees help to move the babies and relieve an aching back.

The heart is pumping at least three pints more blood to flow through additional placentas, and more amniotic fluid is required for more than one baby. Because of this, circulation exercises are important to help prevent swelling of tissues and varicose veins. Plenty of fluids are necessary to stay well hydrated and help prevent preterm labor.

There is not much to do to prevent stretch marks, but using a massage oil over the enlarged abdomen feels good and may help relieve itching.

Low birth weight, prematurity, and the positions in the womb are the most common complications for babies in multiple births, whereas anemia and toxemia are possible complications for the mother. Testing may be performed more frequently in the last trimester to avoid these problems. Ultrasounds are done to keep check on growth and fluid levels, and non-stress tests check heartbeats in reaction to movement. Fetal monitoring from home may be prescribed to watch for preterm labor. While many women carry multiple babies to full term, the average twin pregnancy is 22 days less than normally calculated. Just less than half of all twins and three-fourths of triplets are born early (prior to the 37th week).

At 32 weeks the size of the uterus is about the same as for a singleton at term of 40 weeks. Fatigue sets in earlier and bedrest is a common precaution against a preterm delivery.

The high cesarean birth rate is being challenged for multiples as it is for single babies. Some believe that infant breathing problems may be increased without the stimulation of a vaginal delivery. But many factors play a part in this decision.

Labor for multiples is usually shorter than labor for a single baby, but in some cases a uterus is so stretched that contractions are inefficient and labor is slow. Birth may be easier because the babies tend to be smaller than singletons. Twins' average birth weight (5 pounds, 5 ounces) is about 2 pounds less than the average single baby (7½ pounds). The average difference in birth weight of identical twins is 14 oz. and fraternal twins is 6 oz., but a difference of 2-3 pounds is not extraordinary. Sometimes one twin may absorb more nutrients from a shared placenta than the co-twin.

To give your babies the very best start in life, eat a well-balanced diet with adequate calories and protein; drink lots of water; keep prenatal appointments to check blood and urine, weight gain, and blood pressure; and reduce your stress through time management and relaxation practice. To reduce fear and anxiety, prepare for birth and talk to other parents of multiples. This advice is no different than for other pregnant couples – it's just doubly or triply important!

Multiple Facts

- Twins occur about once in every 90 live births.
- Asian countries have the lowest twinning rate.
- Identical multiples occur when one fertilized egg splits into two or more identical sections which develop separately.
- Fraternal twins are formed from two eggs and two sperm (instead of one which splits) and can look just as similar or different as any siblings.
- Identicals have similar foot and hand prints, but different finger prints.
- About half of identical twins are "mirror" twins. Features such as birthmarks and hair whorls appear on opposite sides of each twin.
- Heaviest twins totalled 27 pounds, 12 ounces. They were born in 1924.
- Lightest living twins weighed 14.8 ounces and 15.5 ounces. They were born in 1994.
- Earliest premature twins to survive were 114 days early. They were born in 1993.

To Be Or Not To Be ... Concerned

At times even normal symptoms of pregnancy such as fatigue, urinary frequency, and back pain are described by the pregnant woman as being different. That feeling alone may indicate a need for medical attention. When visiting a care provider (doctor, nurse, or midwife) the mother will be checked for such things as hypertension, anemia, diabetes, and preeclampsia. The baby will be checked for heart tones, movement, and growth. Take a list of questions or concerns with you – it may save you a "panic call" later.

To assure yourself that all is going well with your pregnancy, it is important to eat well, drink plenty of fluids, nap or relax each day, and spend time "talking" to your baby. After the fifth month of pregnancy, you may want to periodically count your baby's movements (see page 86). Throughout your pregnancy your uterus will contract from time to time. Learn to recognize it so you won't miss the signal if your body warns you of possible premature labor. Early recognition of a preterm labor may prevent a preterm birth, so do not ignore or deny the signals. Learn to feel your contracting uterus by pressing and releasing the muscle with your fingers. Sit comfortably relaxed or lie on your side and begin to "palpate" from the navel, down the center, across to the sides, and back up to the navel. The uterus is contracting if it feels firm to the touch, like touching your forehead.

You can trust your body to give you warning signals if problems arise. You must take the time to listen to those signals and to contact your health care provider when something seems wrong.

Trust your instincts. If you feel that something is not quite right with you or your baby, that is the proper time to be evaluated. On the other hand, remember that many of the "signals" given below can occur normally in pregnancy as well. Some swelling, occasional dizziness, increased discharge or urination, ligament pain, backache, gas pains, "spotting" following sex or examination, pressure from baby's weight, and contractions are all a normal part of pregnancy. It is up to you to determine if what you feel represents a change from your normal experience of pregnancy and if so, seek the advice of your nurse, doctor, or midwife.

Signals of preeclampsia	Signals of infection	Signals of placental or fetal problems
• Persistent or severe headaches • Excessive dizziness • Blurred vision • Excessive swelling • Sudden, rapid weight gain • Protein in urine • Increased blood pressure	• Fever • Vaginal discharge with foul odor • Pain or burning with urination • Decreased amount of urine	• Sharp, persistent abdominal pain • Bleeding from vagina • Decreased fetal activity (less than 10 kicks in 12 hours after the fifth month) • Change in usual pattern of baby's movements

Signals of possible preterm labor	If signals of preterm labor occur	Call your Dr. or midwife immediately if
• Four or more contractions per hour • Low, dull backache • Menstrual-like cramps • Intestinal cramps or diarrhea • Unusual pressure in pelvis, lower back, abdomen, or thighs • Water or large amounts of mucus leaking from the vagina • Red, pink, or brown vaginal discharge • Same signals as for labor, except they occur prior to 37 weeks of pregnancy.	• Stop what you are doing • Empty your bladder • Drink 4 glasses of water (32 oz.) • Lie down on your left side for one hour • Palpate contractions as described above *If you experience four or more contractions per hour before 37 weeks of pregnancy, call your doctor. Often times the signals will weaken or disappear with rest and fluids.*	• Vaginal bleeding occurs • Bag of waters breaks • Uterus contracts 4 or more times per hour before 37 weeks of pregnancy • Major change in baby's movement • Any of your body's signals are of concern to you

Childbirth

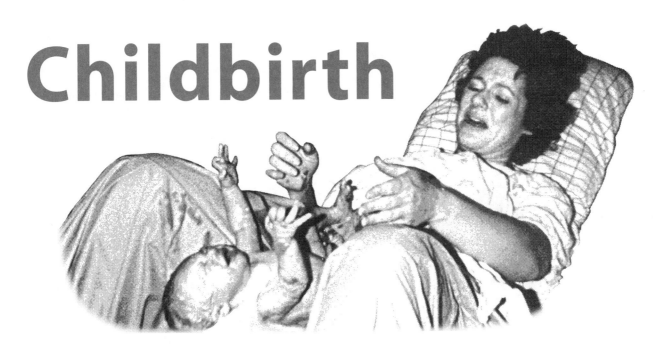

A baby is God's opinion that the world should go on.
Never will a time come when the most marvelous recent
invention is as marvelous as a newborn baby.

Carl Sandburg

Labor Support—Then and Now

Turn of the 20th Century

The way in which pregnancy is acknowledged and the support women have received during labor and birth has varied dramatically since the turn of the 20th century. At that time, the word "pregnancy" was hardly uttered. It was said that a woman was in a "delicate condition," or she was "in the family way." Her birth most often took place in her home, where she was attended by a midwife and surrounded by women. As the century moved on, childbirth began to be viewed as a medical event, rather than as a normal physiological event. Physicians came to replace the midwife, and more births were moved to the hospital. It was then that supportive women and family members were left on the outside and the woman was left to labor alone with the aid of "twilight sleep" (morphine to reduce the pain and scopolamine to remove the memory of pain).

Mid-century

As the negative effects of these drugs and the ensuing instrument deliveries became apparent, Dr. Grantly Dick-Read introduced the idea of educating women about the birth process as a way of controlling childbirth pain. His thoughts were echoed and expanded upon by such people as Drs. Fernand Lamaze, Robert Bradley, and Frederick Leboyer, and women advocates such as Marjorie Karmel and Elisabeth Bing. These people established programs to include the husband as "labor coach" and to allow him to be present as support for his wife during birth. Some men have been eager to assume this role and others extremely reluctant!

The New Millennium

With the turn of the 21st century, the pendulum continues to swing. Pregnancy is spoken of freely, and active pregnant women are seen everywhere. Birth is often viewed on the big screen and on the Internet. The husband or partner is valued for his loving support and encouragement more than for his active instruction. In many regions, women have a choice of birth locations and of people to support them during the birth. A husband, partner, family member, friend, doula, nurse, midwife, and/or physician may have a special role in helping to bring a baby into the world.

A New Option – The Labor Doula

A professional labor assistant, or doula, is gaining popularity as a member of the childbirth team. Whereas physicians, labor nurses, and midwives often must care for more than one laboring woman at a time, a doula may offer continuous support to one woman throughout her labor. A doula does not replace the father in any way, but rather enhances his support of the mother and guides the couple as they labor together. While the father-to-be will most likely wish to be present for the birth of his baby, he does not always feel comfortable being the sole support for his partner. Most often, he has never been present at a birth before and may not have the knowledge and confidence that everything is going just as it should, even when it is. A doula assists the labor nurse in making suggestions for comfort and in giving encouragement and reassurance to the mother or couple through her knowledge and touch. It is her continuous presence, along with her knowledge of and experience with normal birth, that makes her a valuable addition to the birthing team.

Several research studies are summarized in *The Doula Book* by Klaus, Kennell, and Klaus. In these various studies, women who were supported by doulas during labor reported:

- labor and birth as less painful
- feeling more in control of birth
- less anxiety after birth
- feelings of increased self confidence
- a lower incidence of postpartum depression
- increased incidence of breastfeeding at 6 weeks
- improved relationships with their partners

In addition to these very positive perceptions of birth, several studies found that mothers accompanied to labor by a doula had significantly fewer cesarean births, shorter labors, fewer requests for pain medication and anesthesia, less need for oxytocin to stimulate labor, and less need for forceps to assist delivery.

The concept of a doula is not new, but the studies documenting her value are. We are living in the best of times when we can offer the high technology of this century for research, emergencies, or complications while holding on to the high touch skills of women helping women with birth as they did a century ago.

How Long Will Labor Last?

This is the question most frequently asked, but impossible to answer. Each labor and birth is unique. Even different births of the same mother may vary greatly. Many factors affect the length and intensity of labor, such as the following:

Passenger (baby)
- size
- position (facing front, back, or side)
- presentation (head up or down)

Passageway (mom's anatomy)
- cervix (position, degree of effacement and dilation prior to onset of labor, previous surgery or birth, etc.)
- pelvis (size and shape)

Power–strength and efficiency of the contractions

Psyche–mom's fears, anxiety, stress, or confidence

If all these factors are working in Mom's favor at the onset of labor – the baby is a good fit for her pelvis and is facing her back in a head-down position; the cervix has softened, moved forward, and begun to dilate prior to labor; labor contractions are effective; mom's confidence is high and she has good support – then labor may be short. Vary these conditions (as most do) and labor will be longer. Be prepared for anything!

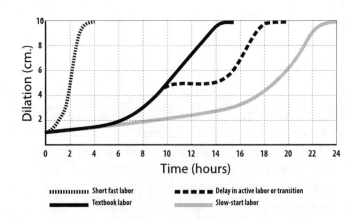

Short fast labor

Textbook labor

Delay in active labor or transition

Slow-start labor

Textbook Labor

According to the labor curve graphed by Dr. E.A. Friedman, the average length of first labors is about 14 hours, and that of subsequent labors about 8 hours. It requires two-thirds of that time to reach 5 cm. dilation. So the longest time is spent in the easiest part of labor when contractions are mildest and farthest apart. Most women can spend much of this time in the comfort of their own homes. You may labor for several hours with no more than twelve minutes worth of contraction each hour (60 second contractions every 5 minutes). The Friedman curve was derived from 500 labors. It took many types of labors to plot an average curve! Remember that your labor will be some variation from the textbook labor.

How to Time Contractions

Duration—beginning to end of one contraction
Frequency —beginning of one contraction to the beginning of the next contraction

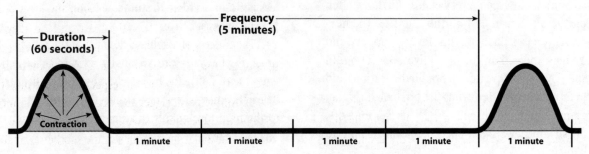

These contractions are coming every 5 minutes and lasting for 60 seconds

Normal Labor Variations

Although most pregnant women expect to have a "textbook" labor and birth, sometimes labor is much shorter or much longer than expected. It may hit a plateau, a delay when very little progress takes place. These variations in labor patterns may require extra patience and coping techniques.

Pre-labor or the Slow-start Labor

Some labors seem to take forever to get started. Contractions may come and go for many hours or even days before the cervix, at long last, begins to open. This type labor is usually more discouraging and tiring than it is painful. Before a cervix can dilate, it must move forward, soften, and thin. This most often takes place in the weeks prior to labor, but sometimes it happens only when the contractions are felt, causing mom to consider herself "in labor" longer. It may seem difficult not to put everything on hold or to rush to the hospital in anticipation of labor, but try to have patience and relax so that you are well rested by the time labor finally "kicks in."

Most of the time, once the cervix dilates to 3-4 centimeters, the rest of the labor proceeds in a normal timely fashion. But it can begin slowly and continue on into a long, slow-but-steady labor to the end.

How to cope with a slow-starting labor:

- Check in with your health care provider if you have any questions about whether or not you need to travel to your birth location.
- If you plan to have a doula attend your labor and birth, stay in contact with her as well as your partner.
- As long as contractions are irregular or continue to start and stop without getting noticeably stronger, continue with your regular activities. Go to work, take in a movie, eat and drink according to your desire, and maintain normal sleep patterns.

Short Fast Labor

While it seems that a very short labor is every woman's dream, it is not always the easiest labor to handle. Contractions come on very suddenly and are usually very intense. It is difficult to maintain control when your mind is expecting early labor contractions but your body has raced almost to 10 cm!

How to cope with rapid onset of hard contractions:

- Get your mind where your body is – be checked to see how far you have dilated.
- Keep eye contact and breathe with your partner.
- If necessary, follow Panic Routine (see page 43).
- Side-lying position may help slow birth.
- Blow through pushing urges.

Delay in Active Labor or Transition

Sometimes labor gets off to a normal start in early labor (0-3cm.), then progress stops instead of accelerating in the later phases. You must take active measures to move off the plateau if this happens. It may be that the size or position of the baby is causing a delay. Position changes and walking may help to move the baby into a better position. If contractions are ineffective, perhaps augmentation of labor will be tried. If labor stalls completely, a cesarean birth may be necessary.

How to cope with a delay in progress:

- Walk!
- Change positions
  - Vertical positions aid gravity
  - Sitting on the toilet may aid the baby's descent
  - Hands and knees may rotate the baby
- Shower or bathe to relax
- Nipple stimulation or other forms of augmentation (oxytocin, enema, rupture of membranes) if birth attendant agrees
- Encouragement and support
- Have patience; allow time

Delay in Second Stage

It is normal for some women to experience a brief time without contractions when the cervix is dilated to 10 centimeters. A British childbirth educator and author, Sheila Kitzinger, calls this the "rest and be thankful" phase. If contractions do not resume within a reasonable amount of time, the laboring woman may want to experiment with upright positions, especially squatting, to see if positioning may trigger the urge to push. If a mother has epidural anesthesia, she may want to decrease or stop the medication. If for any reason the mother is unable to effectively push out her baby, forceps or a vacuum extractor may aid in the birth. Rarely, a cesarean will have to be performed.

How Painful Will Labor Be?

Like the length of labor, pain during childbirth varies from one woman to another and from one birth to another. Personal expectations, cultural and religious beliefs, fear, and anxiety may contribute to the perception of labor pain. However, almost all women in labor will experience the powerful contractions, often referred to as "labor pains," that bring about the birth of a baby. The uterus is the largest and strongest muscle in a woman's body. When it contracts, there is a strong sensation of both pressure and stretching as this powerful muscle pulls back on the cervix to open the door to the birth canal. As the baby moves down the birth canal, additional pressure is exerted on the other internal organs and more stretching occurs. The pain perceived varies from excruciating to mild. In a very few instances a woman will say her labor was not painful at all. The length of labor does not always correlate with the degree of pain. Some short labors are extremely intense and painful while some very lengthy labors are manageable throughout, and vice versa.

There are important differences between the pain of labor and birth and other types of pain that women may experience during their lifetimes.

Purposeful

Anticipated

Intermittent

Normal

Labor Pain is Purposeful

It brings about the birth of a baby. Research studies have shown that laboring women who imagined holding their newborn babies in their arms reported less pain than laboring women who concentrated on other thoughts. Sometimes pain in labor is giving a message to the laboring woman—empty your bladder or change positions to relieve the pressure on your back. Labor pain also triggers the release of stress hormones in the baby which prepare the baby for birth and for adaptation to life outside the uterus. In the mother who has not had pain medication, the release of endorphins is directly correlated with the intensity of the labor contractions. Endorphins are morphine-like substances produced by the body to relieve pain. Long distance runners and athletes striving for peak performances may also experience a purposeful pain and enjoy the "runner's high" produced by endorphins.

Labor Pain is Anticipated

Since you know to expect pain in labor, you are able to prepare yourself ahead of time by learning pain management skills. Pain with an explanation is easier to manage than pain of unknown causes. For most women, labor contractions come in a regular pattern. During labor you will learn the rhythm of your contractions and be able to anticipate when the next one is coming.

Labor Pain is Intermittent

The rest period between contractions is one of the best kept secrets of labor. Labor pain is not continuous as is the pain of kidney stones or an abscessed tooth. Laboring women have a break between contractions to rest and regroup. During the final stages of dilation, the contractions may seem to come one on top of another, but an active partner, nurse, or doula can help you let go of the previous contraction and relax briefly before the next one comes.

Labor Pain is Normal

A woman's body was designed for pregnancy and childbirth. In most cases, labor and birth are normal processes which do not involve illness or injury. Labor contractions are healthy, powerful sensations that push a baby into the outside world. In the same way that exercise enthusiasts, dancers, and athletes push their bodies to perform, many women choose to experience the full normal sensation of labor and birth, even though hard work is required. Deborah Tanzer, a researcher in the psychological aspects of childbirth, found that when women used pain management skills they had learned, they reported peak experiences of joy and fulfillment as well as an improved view of themselves and their capabilities.

Labor pain is normal and natural, but today it is also an option. Look at the Pain Medication Preference Scale on page 98 and decide where you fit on the scale. Then you can discuss your options with your health care provider.

You Will Be Better Able To Deal With Pain If You . . .

- Learn to think positively and overcome fear of birth. Education and information will help to reduce fear of the unknown and fear due to misconceptions. Asking for information and expressing your concerns to knowledgeable people during labor will help to reassure you.

- Establish a support system for yourself. You will want to be surrounded by people who care about you and who will share a positive attitude toward birth with you. Decide what roles you wish for your family, friends, and birth attendants to play. Do not labor alone.

- Select a birth location where you may move freely. Ask if they have rocking chairs, birth balls, and extra pillows. If not, plan to take your own ball and pillows to aid positioning. Upright positions aid labor progress and comfort.

- Practice pain-management skills before birth. Massage, relaxation, and paced breathing can all be used to reduce stress during pregnancy and to cope with contractions during labor. Mastery of these skills will give you confidence in your ability to labor, as well as life-long skills for dealing with tension and stress.

- Try to enter labor well-nourished and well-rested. Everything hurts more when you are tired. Take care of your body's physical and emotional needs in the weeks before the onset of labor.

- Make your labor environment right for you. Adjust the lights. Play music. Relax in a warm tub or shower. Use scented bath oil and/or lotion. Aromatherapists say that lavender promotes relaxation, while jasmine has positive effects on labor progress and comfort. Experiment with scents before labor and take those you like. (See page 84 for suggestions of other things to take.)

- Know your options with regard to medications. What is available to you? What are the risks and benefits of your options? It is your choice whether you wish to work with the pain or ask your care provider to give you relief in the form of medication.

- Remember that pain in labor has a positive purpose. It is pain that you expect, just as an athlete does prior to a major event. Contractions come and go, so more time in labor is spent pain-free than in pain. Giving birth is a normal, natural event in the cycle of life.

For Better or For Worse® **by Lynn Johnston**

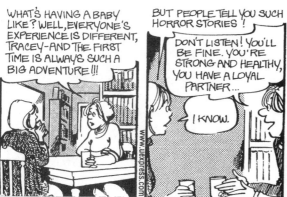
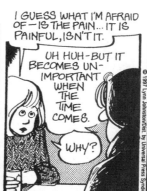
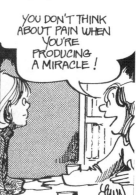

© Lynn Johnston Productions Inc./Distributed by United Feature Syndicate, Inc.

Signs of Labor

Sometimes labor begins before it is really expected, and sometimes it seems that labor will never begin. You may be "teased" by labor's beginning, then stopping, only to begin again on another day. You may be mentally convinced that labor has begun and even have rhythmical contractions coming close together when suddenly, they either stop, or you are examined and your caregiver finds you have made no progress in cervical dilation. Do not despair! You will not be pregnant forever. Some women just experience labor in phases over days or even weeks. What is often called "false labor" is more accurately called "pre-labor." It may be causing the cervix to tilt forward, to soft-en, and to thin—three things that must happen to the cervix before it can open. If you think you are in labor, try the following: walk awhile, relax, shower or bathe, eat foods that are easy to digest, finish packing—then wait until your body tells you that things are "different" enough, or contractions are frequent enough (averaging 60 seconds in length, at five-minute intervals for an hour) to call your caregiver.

Pre-labor signs vary from one woman to the next and from one pregnancy to the next. Any of the following situations may occur as signs of impending labor:

Sign	When It Occurs	What Happens	What Mom Notices	What To Do
Lightening *Engagement*	Two to four weeks before labor	Baby drops or settles into pelvis	Less pressure on stomach and lungs, more pressure on bladder	Wait for more signs of labor
Nesting	A day or two before labor	Impulse to clean or rearrange her "nest"	Sudden burst of energy	Be careful not to become overtired
Show	From hours up to a week before labor	Plug of mucus filling opening of cervix is released, as cervix begins to thin and open	Blood tinged mucous plug	Pack, stay well rested, and be ready when labor begins
Flu-like symptoms *(without fever)*	From hours to days before labor	Nature's way of cleaning out to make way for the baby	Diarrhea, nausea, or mild cramps	Rest, drink fluids, prepare for labor
Backache	Onset of labor and/or during labor	Contracting uterus pulls on lower back	Intermittent backache in time with uterine contractions	Relax, cold packs, heat (bath or shower), massage, positioning
Rupture of membranes	May occur anytime from onset of labor to birth	Tear in amniotic sac causes fluid to leak out	Dampness or trickle of water to gush of fluid from vagina	Call caregiver to report: "*COAT*"–Color, *O*dor, *A*mount, *T*ime; wear a pad or diaper to catch the leaks
Contractions	May occur anytime	Uterine muscles tighten	Weak to strong pressure or pain	Decide if true or false; term or preterm

Pre-labor Contractions

- Generally tighten only portions of the uterus, rarely with back pressure
- Usually of short duration (15-45 seconds)
- Do not increase in intensity
- May not become closer together
- Usually irregular in occurrence
- Changing activity or position may make them stop
- Walking does not make them stronger

True Labor Contractions

- Generally tighten entire uterus and may be felt as back pressure or in low abdomen
- Duration becomes progressively **longer** (up to 60 sec.)
- Become progressively **stronger** in intensity
- Become **closer** together
- Most often become regular in occurrence
- Changing activity or position does not make them stop
- Walking may make them stronger

Stage One: Early Labor

What's Happening

Early labor contractions may start out as far apart as 20 minutes and last only 30 to 45 seconds. If the cervix has not already moved forward, softened, and effaced in preparation for labor, then these important changes in the cervix will take place once labor begins. For the easiest fit, the baby usually faces the mother's side as his head enters the top of the pelvis. During this phase the cervix will completely efface (100%), and dilate to about 3 centimeters. More of the mucous plug, or "show," may be discharged as the cervix opens. Although labor may begin with the breaking of the bag of waters, most often the membranes do not rupture until late in labor. Gradually the contractions become stronger and closer together. As labor progresses to the active phase, regular contractions may be about 5 minutes apart and last up to 60 seconds.

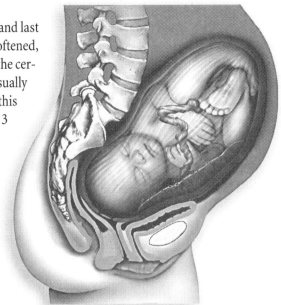

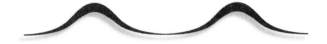

What the Laboring Woman May Feel	What the Laboring Woman Can Do	What the Partner Can Do
• Mild contractions (some women compare to menstrual cramps) • Backache • Mild diarrhea • Excitement • Anticipation • Relief that labor has begun • Happy • Some apprehension	• If labor begins during sleeping hours, try to rest for as long as possible. • Walk! • Change positions frequently, favoring upright positions. • Carry on with normal activities as long as possible, but do not overexert – distract yourself. • Take a warm bath or shower – using a hand-held massager is helpful. • Rest! • Eat and drink lightly. • Try pelvic tilt for backache. • Begin breathing patterns when needed. • RELAX!	• If labor begins during sleeping hours, encourage mom to rest for as long as possible. • Keep mom company – walk with her, play cards, watch TV, etc. • Encourage mom to change positions frequently, favoring upright positions. • Time *some* contractions and keep a written record. • Call birth attendant as he/she has instructed. • Help mom relax! • Massage her back if it aches and suggest comfortable positions. • Tell her how well she is doing. • Put suitcases and pillows in car. • Make yourself a sandwich for goody bag and put in car.

Stage One: Active Labor

What's Happening

During active labor, the contractions continue to increase in intensity and become closer together. They may last 45 to 60 seconds and come as often as every 5 to every 2 minutes. With these stronger contractions, the cervix will continue to open, progressing from about 4 to 7 centimeters. As the baby labors during this phase, he keeps his chin tucked and rotates his body to match the widest part of his head with the widest part of mom's pelvis, so that he will be facing the mother's backbone as he is born.

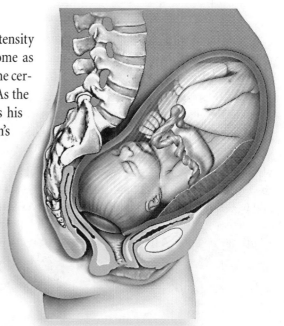

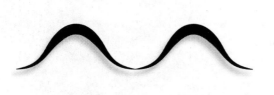

What the Laboring Woman May Feel	What the Laboring Woman Can Do	What the Partner Can Do

• Strong contractions
• Increased backache
• Growing seriousness
• Increasing concentration
• Desire for companionship
• Apprehension
• Uncertain if she can do it
	• Walk if comfortable.
	• Go to hospital/birth center.
	• Change positions often, favoring upright positions.
	• Rock in a rocking chair.
	• Try warm shower and/or bath.
	• Breathe in patterns.
	• Visualize holding the baby in your arms and/or visualize your "special place."
	• During pelvic exams, relax pelvic floor muscles.
		• **SUPPORT** her
		    Supportive environment
		    Urinate at least once an hour
		    Position changes frequently
		    Praise and encouragement
		    Out-of-bed (walk/shower)
		    Relaxation
		    Touch and massage
		• Eliminate distractions in the environment – add to comfort with pillows, dimmed lights, music, etc.
		• Keep lips and mouth moist.
		• Give back massage.
		• Continue to tell her how well she is doing.
		• Change into scrub suit (if requested).

Stage One: Transition

What's Happening

Transition gets its name from the fact that this phase of labor is truly a transition from the powerful and intense contractions that open up the cervix from about 8 to 10 centimeters to the pushing contractions that bring about the birth of the baby. Fortunately for most women, transition is by far the shortest phase of labor, lasting only about 5 to 20 contractions or 10 to 60 minutes. The powerful transition contractions may last 60 to 90 seconds with a break of only one to three minutes between contractions. If the bag of waters has not broken earlier in labor, most often it will break during this phase. The baby has completely turned toward the mother's back and is now ready to begin descending through the birth canal.

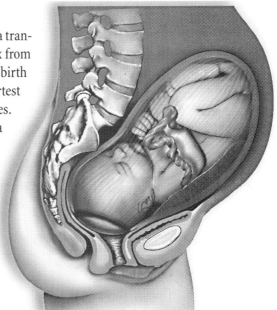

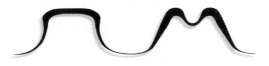

What the Laboring Woman May Feel	What the Laboring Woman Can Do	What the Partner Can Do
• Very intense contractions • Nausea and vomiting • Dozing between contractions • Mood change – irritable • Desire to give up, go home • Hot flashes • Chills and shaking legs • Heavy show • Severe low backache • Possible premature urge to push • Rectal pressure	• Experiment to find your most comfortable position. • Concentrate on the power of the contraction rather than the pain. • Visualize the cervix opening up and the baby moving down. • Take one contraction at a time. • Remember, this is the shortest phase of labor. • Use breathing patterns. • Relax and rest between contractions. • If an urge to push is felt, ask your nurse if small pushes might help labor progress.	• Encourage her to concentrate on the power of the contractions rather than the pain and to use visualization. • Remind her that this is the shortest phase of labor. • Remind her to take one contraction at a time. • Squeeze her hand or give her something to squeeze. • Breathe with her. • Apply counterpressure. • Give her a firm bearhug. • Fan her if she's hot. • Put a cool washrag on her forehead if she is nauseous or hot. • Get extra blankets and massage her legs if she has chills. • Keep lips and mouth moist. • Help her to rest and relax between contractions. • Tell her how great she's doing and that baby will be here soon. • Tell her that you love her.

Stage Two

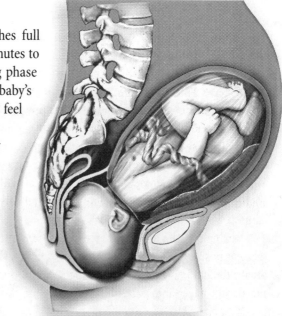

What's Happening

The second stage of labor extends from the time the cervix reaches full dilation to the birth of the baby. This may take anywhere from fifteen minutes to three hours or more. Some women are fortunate to have a brief resting phase between "transition" and "pushing" while the uterus tightens around the baby's body after the head has passed through the cervix. These contractions feel weak to nonexistent compared to the intensity of transition.

Contractions during second stage are usually farther apart than they were in transition, coming about every three to five minutes and lasting about 60 to 90 seconds. Many women find the urge to bear down irresistible as the contraction builds. For most women, the sensations of pushing are much less painful than the contractions of transition.

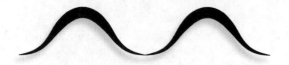

What the Laboring Woman May Feel	What the Laboring Woman Can Do	What the Partner Can Do
• Possible lull – up to 20 minutes while her body rests in preparation for the pushing phase • Almost uncontrollable urge to push • Tremendous back and rectal pressure • "Second wind" of strength to make pushing effort • Pins and needles stretching sensations as baby crowns • Exhaustion between contractions • Relief that she can actively bring about the birth of her baby • Ecstatic sensations as baby is born	• Experiment to find the most comfortable and most productive pushing position: - semi-sitting - side-lying (left) - squatting (widens outlet) - all fours • Relax shoulders, neck, legs, and jaw. • Use spontaneous or directed pushing as explained on page 40. • Relax perineum. • Open your eyes for the birth!	• Help her to find her most comfortable and productive position. • Whisper words of quiet encouragement: "You're doing just fine," "Just like that," "Just perfect." • Encourage her to rest between contractions. • Explain pushing preferences to your nurse so she can work with you. • If she prefers to hold her breath while pushing, remind her to breathe every 6-10 seconds. • Remind her to relax perineum. • Remind her to open her eyes to see the birth.

Stage Three: Delivery of the Placenta

The placenta detaches itself from the uterus and is pushed out through the birth canal in five to twenty minutes.

What the Laboring Woman May Feel	What the Laboring Woman Can Do	What the Partner Can Do
• Mild contractions • Joy • Fatigue • Relief that baby is here	• Gently push as you feel the urge or as instructed by birth attendant. • Do slow paced breathing.	• Give baby to mom to hold or hold baby where mom can see him/her.

Breathing Strategies for Labor

Breathing Awareness

Before practicing the paced breathing techniques, become aware of your normal breathing. Place your hand on your upper chest. Feel the movement as you inhale and exhale. Move your hand to the lower curve of your abdomen; again, feel the movement. Your partner may place hands in various positions on your back (at the tailbone, the waist, the shoulder-blades, then at the top of the shoulders). Focus your attention on the warmth and pressure of touch and breathe towards it. Practicing this will better enable you to find a comfortable level of breathing in labor.

During practice and in labor – assume a comfortable, relaxed position; select a focal point; take a cleansing breath to begin and end each contraction; and breathe to the depth, pace, and pattern that suits your individual needs. Specific rates for the breathing patterns should be individualized for each person. Your partner should count the number of breaths you normally take in a one-minute period to get your baseline. This baseline will determine the rates recommended.

Mom's baseline is _____ breaths per minute.

Partner's baseline is _____ breaths per minute.

Slow Paced Breathing

This is a slow breathing pattern in which the chest and abdomen gently expand on inhalation and relax on exhalation. Breathing in and out through the nose is natural for most people. However, throughout labor, you should breathe in whatever way is most comfortable for you – in and out through the nose; in through the nose and out through the mouth; or in and out through the mouth. The rate for slow paced breathing should be about half that of your normal breathing rate. This relaxed pattern is used by some women throughout their labors.

Modified Paced Breathing

Paced breathing can be modified to accommodate the urge to breathe faster as the contraction becomes more intense. The rate may increase to as much as twice your baseline. However, your partner should help you to pace yourself as breathing is more relaxed at slower rates. Breathing through your mouth may be preferred at times.

Strategies to Accompany Paced Breathing

Visualize scenes such as
- an ocean wave slowly rolling in as you inhale; slowly rolling out as you exhale.
- being surrounded by your favorite relaxing color and breathing in that color to spread its relaxing effects to all of your body; then breathing out a color of tension.
- the soft petals of a flower gradually opening up as the morning sun strikes them.
- (only when you are in labor) your cervix opening, opening, opening to the full 10 centimeters so that the baby can enter the birth canal.

Repeat rhythmical phrases such as
- "Breathe in for my baby, breathe out tension."
- "Breathe in energy, blow away pain."

Count
- to a designated number such as 4 or 5 as you inhale; do the same as you exhale.
- your own pattern by inhaling and exhaling a designated number of times; then substitute a soft blow or "puh" for the exhalation (example: 3 to 1 pattern – inhale, exhale; inhale, exhale; inhale, exhale; inhale, soft blow or "puh"). The labor partner can change the pattern (example: 3 to 1 pattern, then 2 to 1 or 4 to 1 pattern) during the contraction by signaling with his fingers or voice which pattern the laboring mother should use (see page 95).

Whisper words or syllables on exhalation such as
- "hee" or "huh." (Keep mouth, lips, and jaw relaxed.)
- "hee" or "huh" a certain number of times, then give a soft blow or "puh." (Example: "hee, hee, blow.")

Combine
- slow and modified paced breathing by using slow paced at the beginning and end of the contraction, and modified only over the more difficult peak of the contraction.
- imagery and counting such as visualizing a room full of lighted candles and counting them as you blow them out.
- any of the strategies above.

Pushing Techniques for Birth

It is not always easy to tell just when second stage begins. Some women experience a lull after the cervix has dilated to ten centimeters. This rest period may allow the baby to descend deeper into the pelvis and may help the laboring woman to gather strength for bearing-down efforts. Other women may feel an urge to push before the cervix is completely dilated. There are times when small, natural pushes may aid labor progress, and other times when active pushing should be delayed.

Spontaneous Pushing

Spontaneous pushing is used when the mother feels strong pushing urges. She responds by bearing down according to what she is feeling. Rather than counting or loudly calling out encouragement, her support team remains silent or whispers quiet words of support and encouragement.

- Experiment to find the position most comfortable and efficient for you. A supported squat position may increase the urge to push.
- Remember – you are using only your abdominal (voluntary) and uterine (involuntary) muscles for pushing, so position yourself so you can relax the muscles in your arms, shoulders, legs, and face.
- Use any breathing pattern you like as the contraction builds. When you feel the urge to bear down, tune in to your body and push as you feel the need. Rest or take another deep breath as needed.
- You may make "birthing" or "grunting" sounds while slowly exhaling with the bearing-down effort.
- Three to five efforts are usually made across the peak of each contraction, as your body commands.

Directed Pushing

Directed pushing is used if the mother is anesthetized, if baby's descent is too slow, or if hospital routine dictates. The anesthetized mother may not be directed to push until the baby has descended to a plus-one station, or perhaps until the head is visible.

- Begin each contraction with a cleansing breath. As the contraction builds, breathe in and out two more times.

- On the third breath in, hold your breath, but not for more than six seconds at a time (a fast count to ten). After your labor partner has counted to ten, blow out quickly and take another breath, hold and push. Repeat until the contraction subsides. This will usually be three or four directed efforts.
- When the contraction is over, take a cleansing breath and rest.

Strategies to consider

- If directed by your caregiver to avoid pushing, it may be necessary to blow or "puff" repeatedly when you feel your body starting to push.
- Your birth attendant may do perineal massage to help the tissues stretch. Push into his or her touch while releasing the pelvic floor muscles. Practicing perineal massage ahead of time may help. Think or say – "Open, oooopen!"
- If you feel you are not pushing effectively, ask your labor attendant to put a gloved hand or a warm compress on your perineum so you can feel the direction to push. A mirror placed so you can watch your progress when you push may also encourage and direct you.
- Try to imagine what is happening inside your body by visualizing your baby moving down the birth canal.
- When you feel a burning, stretching sensation, you will know your baby's birth is near. Try to release the pelvic floor muscles and concentrate on your baby.
- Partners can provide support by whispering encouraging phrases such as, "Just like that," "Good work," and "The baby's almost here."

Positions for Second Stage

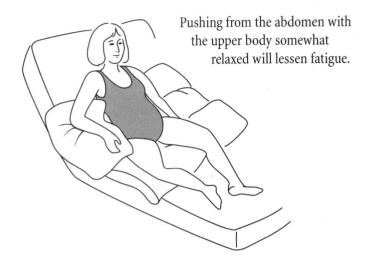

Pushing from the abdomen with the upper body somewhat relaxed will lessen fatigue.

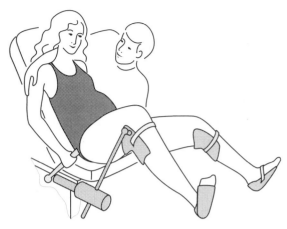

Semi-sitting is the most common position for birth and is usually the position of choice if an epidural block is in place. Stirrups may or may not be used.

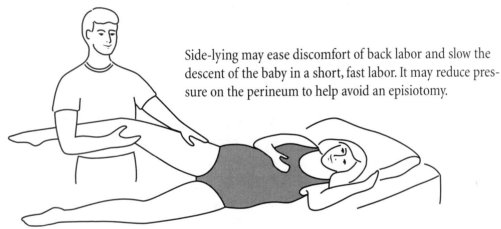

Side-lying may ease discomfort of back labor and slow the descent of the baby in a short, fast labor. It may reduce pressure on the perineum to help avoid an episiotomy.

Being on hands and knees may help rotate a baby from the posterior to the anterior position and relieve pressure on mom's back.

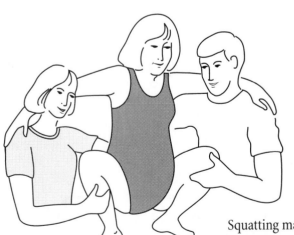

Squatting may help to widen the pelvic outlet and encourage a large baby to come down.

Possible Challenges of Labor

Challenge	Solution
Nausea	• Take slow, deep breaths. • Lie on left side or try sitting up. • Apply cool washrag to face. • Remember, nausea can be a sign of transition.
Chills/shakes	• Put on socks. • Add warm blankets and/or heat pack. • Use concentration and focal point. • Contract, then release all muscles. • Try other relaxation techniques such as visual imagery. • Do friction rub. • Partner give her a bearhug.
Leg cramps	• Partner place heel of affected leg in palm of his hand and use arm to gently push ball of foot toward mom's head. • Do foot twirls. • Apply warm blankets or compresses.

Back labor	• Change mother's position – get the baby off her spine (see pgs. 20-21)
	   – Side-lying with uterus tilted toward bed, pillow between knees
	   – Sitting up with back rounded
	   – Sitting up on side of bed with arms supported on bedside table
	   – All fours (on floor or over back of bed)
	• Try movement to encourage baby to rotate to an anterior position
	   – Pelvic tilt on all fours
	   – Walking up and down stairs
	   – Standing or kneeling lunge
	• Apply counterpressure
	   – Partner's hand
	   – Massage toy, small paint roller, or tennis balls in a sock
	• Apply heat or cold
	   – Warm shower or bath
	   – Tupperware rolling pin filled with ice or hot water
	   – Ice packs or cold compresses
	   – Heating pad/hot water bottle, microwave heat pack

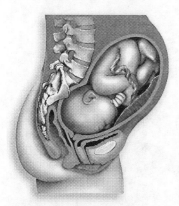

Baby in posterior position puts pressure on spine

To make a reusable heat pack: Put 3 cups of uncooked rice in a cotton tube sock. Sew or tie the top closed. Microwave for 2 to 3 minutes for warm, moist heat.

What To Do If The Laboring Woman Panics

Many women ride every contraction of their labor with seeming ease and poise. However, many more feel that some contractions overwhelm them – that they "lose control" or "panic" and call out for help. The support person can help prevent this panic in some instances or help the mother regain control by being familiar with the "Panic Routine."

Pre-Panic Signals	Role of Partner
Restless or agitated body movements	Observe tension, and: • Stroke it away with both touch and verbal signals ("Release where I touch you, release to my hands.") • Apply back pressure if needed. • Talk it away ("Uncurl your toes," "I'll hold your hand," "Take a cleansing breath.") • Use key phrases from your "special place" to encourage relaxation.
Unrhythmical, loud, or irregular breathing	Breathe with her. Start with her pace and slow it if necessary.
Loss of focal point *Eyes darting about or head moving side to side*	Keep your face close to hers. "Look at me."
Verbally giving up *"I can't do this anymore!"*	This is a request for support. Acknowledge her pain. Reassure her, praise her, take charge. Try to get her to focus on the power of the contraction rather than the pain. See if you can get her to visualize the cervix opening up and the baby moving down. Use as much of the "Panic Routine" as needed.

Panic Routine for Labor Partner

1. *Establish eye-to-eye contact* – Position yourself so that your face is directly in front of hers. You may need to stand up.

2. *Hold her firmly* – Take either her hands, shoulders, or face in your hands to focus her attention on you. If she pulls away from you, do not give up; re-establish physical contact.

3. *Breathe with her* – Tell her to breathe with you. Breathe loudly or use words or blows so that she can easily follow you. Begin at her pace and guide her to slower, quieter breaths as she follows you.

4. *Reassure her* – After the contraction is over, assure her that you will be there to help her with each contraction. Remind her that each contraction brings her closer to the birth of the baby. Words of encouragement and support from you, the nurse, and your caregiver can make all the difference in the world.

Childbirth Choices

Many articles have been written about routine medical procedures and current trends in childbirth. Some procedures that were "routine" several years ago are now done on an "as needed" basis. Policies vary from one hospital to another, and individual caregivers' practices also differ. Some pregnant women feel most comfortable with the idea of a high-tech birth, while others want as "natural" an experience as possible. It is important to think about the type of birth you would like ahead of time, and to discuss your preferences with your health care provider. It is also important to understand that labor and birth sometimes do not go as expected. Understanding the benefits and risks of common procedures and medications will help you to make informed decisions. Remaining flexible will help you to work positively with your particular labor and birth.

Induction

Induction is the process of starting labor by artificial means. It should not be done as a convenience for the pregnant woman or the doctor, but should only be performed when medically indicated. Prolonged rupture of the membranes without contractions, a pregnancy that has lasted longer than 42 weeks, or toxemia in the mother are all possible medical reasons for induction. According to the American College of Obstetricians and Gynecologists (ACOG), suspecting even a very large baby is not a medical indication for induction. Research studies have shown that inducing for this increases, rather than decreases, the likelihood of cesarean birth.

Labor may be induced by the application of a prostaglandin gel or other medications to stimulate ripening of the cervix, by artificially rupturing the membranes (amniotomy), or by the intravenous (IV) administration of oxytocin (Pitocin). Either of these latter methods of induction might also be used to augment a stalled labor if such things as changing position, walking, or nipple stimulation are ineffective. If oxytocin is used, labor is usually monitored continuously with an electronic fetal heart monitor to assure that the baby is tolerating the labor without undue stress. Induced contractions are often stronger and/or more frequent than natural contractions, requiring additional coping techniques.

Non-Stress Test, Biophysical Profile, and Stress Test

Before inducing labor, some physicians perform a non-stress or a stress test. During a non-stress test, an external fetal monitor is attached to the mother's abdomen. The doctor studies the baby's heartbeat when the baby is moving. If the heartbeat is fine, the mother is allowed to go home and wait (usually another week) for labor to begin on its own. If the heartbeat indicates that the baby should be born as soon as possible, then labor is induced or a cesarean birth occurs. For mothers at risk for a complicated pregnancy, a biophysical profile combines the nonstress test and ultrasound. The baby's breathing movements, muscle tone, body movement, and the amount of amniotic fluid are evaluated during the biophysical profile. During a stress test, contractions are induced with oxytocin while the baby's heartbeat is monitored with an external electronic fetal monitor. If the heartbeat appears strong and healthy, the mother is allowed to go home and wait (usually a week) for labor to begin spontaneously. If the test indicates that the baby should be born very soon, then the oxytocin is continued and/or increased for an induction, or a cesarean birth occurs.

Fluids by Mouth/Intravenous Infusion (IV)

In a long labor, women need fluids in order to prevent dehydration. In many hospitals and birth centers, laboring women are encouraged to take fluids such as ice chips, popsicles, water, and other clear liquids by mouth, while others require fluids by IV. Giving fluids through a plastic tube inserted into a vein in the hand or arm is called an IV. An IV may be used to provide an easy route for the administration of medication or for emergency procedures. It may be uncomfortable or more difficult to move around with an IV in place, but with a rolling IV pole, it is still possible to walk, taking it along. It may be possible to delay the start of a required IV until near the beginning of second stage, when most women stay in bed, or to substitute a heparin lock which holds a vein open without the attachment to an IV bag and pole. If your labor is induced with oxytocin or if you choose to have epidural anesthesia, an IV will be necessary.

Monitoring Fetal Heart Tones

According to the American College of Obstetricians and Gynecologists (ACOG) and the Association of Women's Health, Obstetric, and Neonatal Nurses (AWHONN), there are several safe and effective ways to monitor the baby's heartbeat during labor.

Caregivers may use a specially designed stethoscope

(fetoscope) or a hand-held electronic device (Doppler) to listen to the baby's heartbeat on a regular schedule. With these types of intermittent monitoring, the laboring woman is free to walk, slow dance, use a birth ball or rocking chair, and change positions often. She can also easily take a warm bath or shower. Intermittent monitoring does require the frequent presence of the labor nurse.

Electronic fetal heart monitoring is a method of measuring and recording the baby's heartbeat in relation to the mother's uterine contractions. A monitor may be applied either externally by two belts around the mother's abdomen or internally through the vagina to the baby's scalp and to the uterus. The internal monitor is more accurate and comfortable for the woman, but membranes must be ruptured for its use. Monitor cords limit movement, but a woman is not always confined to bed. She may sit in a rocking chair, use a birth ball, or stand and sway nearby the monitor. Some external fetal monitor belts are waterproof, so that the laboring woman can take a bath or shower while being monitored. The external monitor may be removed after a baseline is obtained so that the mother can walk. Telemetry, a way of monitoring without cords attached to the monitor, is available at some hospitals.

For most mothers, continuous monitoring is not required unless oxytocin or an epidural is used. In some high risk pregnancies, it may be beneficial to have a constant reading on the condition of the baby throughout labor. A study by Dr. Kenneth Leveno, reported in *The New England Journal of Medicine*, concluded that "not all pregnancies, and particularly not those considered at low risk of perinatal complications, need continuous electronic fetal monitoring during labor."

Amniotomy

Breaking the bag of waters by using an amnihook is called an amniotomy. This is sometimes done to see the color of the amniotic fluid (meconium-stained fluid may indicate fetal distress) or to induce or augment labor. Contractions may increase in frequency and intensity following amniotomy, thereby possibly shortening some labors. Intact, the bag of waters cushions the baby's head and reduces the chance of bacteria reaching the baby and the uterine cavity. Once the membranes are ruptured, either on their own or by amniotomy, many healthcare providers feel that the baby should be born within 24 hours to reduce the chance of infection.

Episiotomy

An episiotomy is a surgical incision of the perineum made to enlarge the vaginal opening at the time of birth. This makes more room for the birth of a large baby or for the use of forceps. A local anesthetic is given so that the episiotomy repair is not painful, but most women report some pain after the anesthetic wears off. The length of recovery time varies among women. Some caregivers believe that it may help to avoid an episiotomy if massage is used to help stretch the perineal tissues during pregnancy or during birth. This massage may slightly prolong the delivery by giving time for the perineum to stretch, but the new mother will not have to cope with the pain from an episiotomy. The position for delivery, the elasticity of the perineum, and the size of the baby determine whether or not an episiotomy is necessary. The American College of Obstetricians and Gynecologists (ACOG) does not recommend routine use of episiotomies.

Forceps/Vacuum Extractor

Forceps or a vacuum extractor (suction device) may be used to help during a difficult delivery. Both delivery tools are used to speed up second stage if the baby needs to be delivered quickly or if the mother can't push effectively due to anesthesia, exhaustion, or the size of the baby. An episiotomy is required when forceps are used. Forceps may cause bruises on the baby, which generally fade in about 48 hours. The vacuum extractor may cause a little swelling, but this too soon disappears.

Circumcision

Circumcision is the surgical removal of all or part of the foreskin of the penis. Sometimes it is done for religious reasons, as in the Jewish faith. In the hospital setting, it is not done automatically on all boys, but is an operative procedure which requires the informed, signed consent of the parents. In 1999, the American Academy of Pediatrics (AAP) stated that the benefits of circumcision are not significant enough for the AAP to recommend circumcision for all newborn baby boys. Instead, they recommend that parents discuss the benefits and risks of circumcision with their baby's health care provider, and then make an informed decision about what is in the best interest of their child. The AAP also states that if parents decide to circumcize their infant, it is essential that pain relief be provided.

Rooming-in

Rooming-in encourages a new family to get acquainted while in the hospital. The baby spends all or part of the day and night in the mother's room. Medical staff are near to answer questions and to help the new parents gain confidence in caring for their baby before they go home.

Having the baby near the mother for frequent feedings helps get breastfeeding off to a good start. Some hospitals offer daytime rooming-in only, but many also offer it at night, if desired.

Management of Labor Pain

Sensations of uterine contractions have been described by laboring women as anything from "pressure" to "intense pain." Some women do not realize they are having contractions until birth is about to occur, yet others report labor pain for days before birth. Just as women's perceptions of labor pain vary, so do women's choices about pain management. Your choices regarding comfort measures and pain medications may depend upon the intensity and length of your labor; your own fears, concerns, and plans; the options available at your birth location; and the support you receive during labor.

Your own natural resources and education may provide the relief you need. Frequent position changes and movements such as walking, slow dancing, and doing the pelvic tilt on all fours may reduce pain, as well as help the baby to descend. Warm baths and showers, massage, relaxation and paced breathing techniques along with the body's endorphins (morphine-like pain inhibitors which our bodies produce in high levels during an unmedicated labor) allow many women to cope with labor pain and to experience positive sensations of birth.

Studies have shown that the presence of a doula for physical and emotional labor support has significantly decreased the length of labor and the pain perceived.

Narcotics and tranquilizers (pages 48-49) reduce pain and tension, whereas regional anesthetics (spinal and epidural blocks) numb the sensations of contractions and birth. Various medications provide pain relief for women who do not want to cope with the pain of contractions. However, no medication is without possible side effects; therefore any medication should be used carefully and with informed consent.

Epidural Anesthesia
Keith J. Reisler, M.D.

Epidural anesthesia refers to a numbing of the lower half of the body for pain relief during labor, delivery, or cesarean birth. An epidural is given with the patient on her side or sitting up. First, an IV is started in the vein of the hand or arm, and fluid is administered. A small area of skin on the lower back is numbed with local anesthesia. A needle is then placed through this area to the epidural space which is located outside the spinal sheath. A small plastic catheter is placed through the needle while the needle is withdrawn. The catheter is taped to the back, with one end remaining in the epidural space and the other end attached to the syringe of anesthetic medicine, which can then be injected into the epidural space. The catheter remains in place throughout labor and birth, during which time small amounts of anesthetic can be injected intermittently, either manually or by an electric pump.

The amount of numbing depends on the drug and dose used. The medicine injected will affect the nerve fibers as they pass from the spinal column to the lower body. This will allow pain relief from uterine contractions and during vaginal delivery. Pain relief may vary from complete to partial. During a cesarean birth, higher doses of medicine are used. The motor fibers are also numbed with a traditional epidural, making movement of the legs difficult and walking impossible. Recently narcotic medications have been injected alone or in combination with these numbing medications. These narcotic epidurals or "walking epidurals" give less numbing, allowing greater movement and possible walking. However, the pain relief experienced will usually not be as great as with the traditional epidural. Narcotic epidurals are not available in all hospitals.

Epidural anesthesia is more likely to slow labor if given prior to the active phase. Experts do not agree as to whether epidural anesthesia may increase the cesarean rate, especially when given early in the labor. Some studies suggests that receiving epidural anesthesia prior to 5 cm. of dilatation may increase the rate of cesarean delivery in women having their first baby. Epidural anesthesia slows the second stage of labor ("pushing stage"), since bearing down is more difficult. This will increase the need for suction devices or forceps to assist the delivery.

Epidural block can have certain side effects. The mother's blood pressure may drop, which can usually be avoided by administering approximately a pint of IV fluid before the injection. If this does happen, the baby's heart rate may slow. Other complications are rare. If the covering of the spinal cord is punctured when the needle is placed, the mother may develop a severe headache which may last a few days. If the dose of numbing medication used for epidural analgesia enters the spinal fluid or a vein around the epidural space, other serious complications may develop, such as difficulty breathing or rarely seizures. All of these events are rare in experienced hands (also see page 49).

Emergency Birth

The most important thing to remember about emergency deliveries is that they are almost always very fast, easy, and uncomplicated. The attendant needs to do little more than "catch the baby."

1. If there seems to be no way to make it to the hospital, call 911 or an ambulance so that trained personnel are on their way. If you are enroute to the hospital or birth center when birth becomes imminent, trained paramedics may be available at the nearest fire station.

2. Try to help the mother relax and release all muscle groups.

3. Encourage the mother to assume the most comfortable position for delivery.

4. Clean newspapers can be placed underneath the mother to act as absorbent padding. A clean sheet should be placed over the newspapers.

5. The attendant should wash his or her hands up to the elbows for about four minutes or use an alcohol-based hand sanitizer.

6. As the baby is crowning, many mothers have a tendency to hold back on their pushing efforts for fear of "splitting open" their perineum. This holding back should definitely be encouraged. Whether or not the mother has this tendency, she should be instructed to blow while the head is being delivered so that she does not contribute to the involuntary pushing efforts of the uterus. In addition, the attendant should place one hand on the baby's head and apply very gentle counter-pressure to the head as it is emerging so that it is born in a very slow, controlled manner. This will help to minimize possible harm to the baby and to the mother's perineum.

7. As soon as the head is born, the attendant should check to see if the amniotic sac is still intact around the baby. If it is, there will be a cellophane-like covering over the baby. Break this with any clean, sharp item and gently wipe the baby's face. If the cord is around the baby's neck, slip it over the head. *Do not pull on the baby in order to deliver the rest of the body.*

8. The baby's shoulders will probably be delivered during the next contraction or two. The attendant should support the baby's head and encourage the mother to push as hard as she can to aid in the expulsion of the shoulders. Once the shoulders are delivered, the rest of the baby will slip out very quickly.

9. Once the baby is fully delivered, hold the baby with the head lower than its body so that any fluids or mucus swallowed during delivery will drain out. With your fingers, gently wipe out any mucus in the baby's mouth. Wrap a clean towel or blanket around the baby and place him between the mother's legs for warmth.

10. *Do not attempt to cut the cord.* Wait until trained personnel arrive or until you can get mother and baby to the hospital.

11. If the cord is long enough to allow, put the baby to the mother's breast. The skin-to-skin contact will help keep the baby warm and the baby's suckling will help the placenta to detach from the wall of the uterus.

12. *Do not pull on the cord to help deliver the placenta.* The placenta will come out in its own good time, or its delivery can wait until you get to the hospital. If the placenta is delivered at home, be sure to save it to take to the hospital so the doctor can examine it. If the baby is not already at the mother's breast, be sure to put the baby immediately to breast as soon as the placenta is delivered. The baby's suckling will stimulate the uterus to contract and help to prevent possible dangerous bleeding (normal blood loss following childbirth is less than two cups).

13. Use blankets to keep mother and baby warm and to help mother's "shakes."

CONGRATULATIONS!

Medications Available During Labor and Birth

STAGE ONE LABOR – Systemic drugs (affect the whole body)

Type of Drug	How Given/When Given	Duration	Purpose	Possible Effects on Mom	Possible Effects on Baby	Possible Effects on Labor
Barbiturates (*sleeping pills*) Seconal Nembutal Amytal	By mouth, IM (into muscle), or IV (into vein). IM medication crosses placenta within 5 minutes; IV within 1 minute Generally given only in very early labor	Seconal: 4-6 hrs Nembutal: 4-6 hrs Amytal: 7-8 hrs	• Often given to distinguish true labor contractions from pre-labor contractions • To promote rest and relaxation • Have no effect on pain	• Drowsiness • More difficult to focus during contractions • Nausea • Large doses: hypotension (low blood pressure), decreased pulse rate, and disorientation	• Respiratory depression • Decreased responsiveness • Decreased sucking ability • Hypotonia (decreased muscle tone) *Most pronounced if given within 4 hours of birth*	None known
Analgesics/Narcotics Demerol Nubain Stadol Sublimaze	Demerol: IM or IV Nubain: sub-Q (injected just under skin), IM or IV Stadol: IM or IV Sublimaze: IM or IV *Note: Some analgesics/narcotics are now being administered through the epidural catheter.* Generally given only in active labor	Demerol: 2-3 hrs Nubain: 3-6 hrs Stadol: 3-4 hrs Sublimaze: 1-2 hrs	• To "take the edge off" the pain • To raise the pain threshold • To reduce pain (central nervous system depressant)	• Drowsiness • Disorientation • More difficult to focus during contractions • Hypotension • Nausea/vomiting • Dry mouth • Dizziness • IV: respiratory depression	• Respiratory depression • "Sleepy" baby • Decreased sucking ability *Most pronounced if given within 1 to 3 hours of birth*	• Can slow down labor • Need for additional medical procedures (continuous monitoring of fetal heart rate, IV)
Tranquilizers Valium Phenergan Vistaril Largon	IM or IV	Valium IM: 2-3 hrs Valium IV: 1-1½ hrs Phenergan: 6-8 hr Vistaril: 4-6 hrs Largon: 3 hrs	• To reduce tension and anxiety • To relieve nausea • To relax muscles • To enhance effects of narcotics	• Drowsiness • Difficulty concentrating • Dry mouth • Hypotension	• "Sleepy" baby • Decreased responsiveness • Slow adaptation to feeding	None known

STAGE ONE LABOR – Regional Anesthetics (only affect one portion of the body)

Type of Drug	How Given/When Given	Duration	Purpose	Possible Effects on Mom	Possible Effects on Baby	Possible Effects on Labor
Paracervical – one of the "caine" drugs is used	Given in active labor while lying on back. Needle inserted into nerve trunks of cervix via vagina.	Takes effect in 3-4 minutes and lasts 1-2 hrs; can be repeated until about 8 cm	To block uterine pain	None known	Bradycardia (slow heart rate)	Can slow down contractions

Type of Drug	How Given/When Given	Duration	Purpose	Possible Effects on Mom	Possible Effects on Baby	Possible Effects on Labor
Epidural • "caine" drug (such as Fentanyl) • narcotic (such as Fentanyl) • "caine" drug + narcotic	Given in active labor while sidelying or sitting. Needle introduced into epidural space (not spinal fluid) and catheter inserted. Catheter left in place for continuous administration or in case additional medication is needed.	Takes about 30 minutes to administer. Duration depends on drug used and method of administration (continuous or intermittent)	• To relieve painful sensations of contractions, birth, and episiotomy repair • To allow mom to be awake and alert • Can be used for forceps/cesareans	• Hypotension (low blood pressure). • Incomplete coverage • 3% failure rate for epidural • Fever • Need for urinary catheter • Increased incidence of 3rd & 4th degree perineal lacerations	• Hypotension in mom can cause drop in fetal heart rate • Septic workup if mom has fever • More research needed regarding possible subtle behavioral alterations	• IV fluids and continuous electronic fetal heart rate monitoring required • Increased length of labor • Increased need for oxytocin augmentation • Higher incidence of operative vaginal deliveries (vaccuum, forceps)
Intrathecal Narcotics (within spinal canal) Sufentanil Fentanyl Demerol Morphine	During active labor, a narcotic is injected into the subarachnoid space (space containing the spinal fluid) Utilizes a smaller needle than used for epidural analgesia	• 90-120 minutes • May be repeated, but offers much shorter period of pain relief	• For rapid onset of pain relief • No effect on motor function • May not provide adequate pain relief for second stage (see combined spinal-epidural)	• May retain mobility • Able to feel urge to push • May cause itching, nausea, vomiting, urinary retention, hypotension, and spinal headaches (1-2%), respiratory depression	Some studies have shown fetal heart rate abnormalities, especially bradycardia (slow heart rate), while other studies have not	• IV fluids and continuous electronic fetal heart rate monitoring required • Morphine may prolong labor

Combined spinal-epidural analgesia is given in active labor and is intended to continue through birth. When the intrathecal narcotic is given, an epidural catheter is placed to administer anesthetics after the intrathecal dose wears off. Although this procedure combines the effects of both intrathecal narcotics and epidural analgesia, the laboring woman will not be mobile and may not feel the urge to push.

STAGE II – Birth of the baby

a. Systemic drugs are not recommended because of possible adverse effects on baby when given near the time of birth.

b. Regional anesthetics (in addition to epidural, intrathecal narcotics, or combined spinal-epidural analgesia)

Type of Drug	How Given	Duration	Purpose	Possible Effects on Mom	Possible Effects on Baby	Possible Effects on Labor
Local – one of the "caine" drugs	Injection into perineum immediately prior to episiotomy or after birth for repair	Takes effect in 5 minutes and lasts 20 minutes	Anesthesia for episiotomy and episiotomy repair	None	None	None
Pudendal Block - one of the "caine" drugs	Injection into pudendal nerves via vagina immediately prior to birth or after birth for repair	Takes effect in 2-3 minutes and lasts 1 hour	• Anesthesia for vagina and perineum • Used for forceps	Eliminates "stretching" sensations	None, except with preexisting fetal distress	• Partial loss of urge to push • Relaxation of perineum
Spinal/Saddle. Spinal provides anesthesia from breasts down. *Saddle* effects those parts which rest on a saddle.	Injection into spinal fluid given side-lying or sitting bent over with back bowed	Takes effect in 3-5 minutes and lasts 1½ - 2 hours	• Complete anesthesia for contractions, birth, repair • To allow mom to be awake and alert • Can be used for forceps and cesarean deliveries	• Hypotension • Spinal headache • Bladder atony (need for catheter)	• Hypotension in mom can cause drop in fetal heart rate • More research needed regarding possible subtle behavioral alterations	• Contractions may be stopped • Urge to push is lost • Forceps needed

Are All Cesareans Necessary?

Data from the National Center for Health Statistics (NCHS) of the Centers for Disease Control and Prevention (CDC) show that the overall cesarean rate in the United States steadily increased from 5.5 % in 1970 to a peak of 24.7% in 1988 (nearly 1 in 4 births). During these years of increased surgical births, it was found that there was no overall improvement in the health of mother or baby and that surgery indeed presented an increased risk of childbirth complications. One of the Healthy People Year 2000 objectives was to reduce the overall cesarean rate to 15% and the primary (first time) cesarean rate to 12 or fewer per 100 deliveries. The cesarean birth rate dropped slowly, starting in the early 1990's, to a low of 20.7% in 1996, but has recently started to rise again, with the overall rate for 2001 being 24.4%. It is the responsibility, not only of physicians, but also of pregnant women to help lower the cesarean rate. The following information may help you give yourself the best possible chance to avoid an unnecessary cesarean:

- Maintain good nutrition to allow your body a fair start into labor.
- Obtain good prenatal care.
- Discuss policies and criteria for cesarean deliveries and vaginal birth after cesarean (VBAC) with your doctor or midwife.
- Understand the use, benefits, and risks of:
  - obstetrical drugs and anesthesia;
  - induction of labor (by artificial rupture of membranes, use of IV oxytocin, or prostaglandins);
  - the electronic fetal heart monitor;
  - x-ray pelvimetry and ultrasound.
- In many parts of the county, a baby in a breech or transverse presentation is most often delivered by cesarean. However, more and more physicians are successfully rotating babies to a head-down position by a technique called external version. Discuss this with your doctor. If your baby is in a breech presentation at 32 weeks, with your doctor's permission, try *Rotating A Breech* (see below).

When labor begins, the prepared couple has the advantage of knowing how to give their labor the optimum chance of progressing. Remember these points:

- Avoid induction of labor unless medically indicated.
- Avoid epidural anesthesia in early labor. If given, request the medication be decreased or turned off if labor stops progressing or when second stage is reached (so that you can push more effectively).
- Walk through as much of labor as you can.
- Change position frequently; avoid lying flat. If available, use the rocking chair or birth ball.
- Urinate every hour.
- Relax – especially if labor slows. Try all techniques and give your body time. If available, a warm bath or shower can especially aid relaxation.
- Partner and medical team must give encouragement – essential with a slow labor.
- In second stage, push with your body's urge. Try squatting if you have no natural urge-to-push or if the baby remains "high."

There are occasions when, regardless of what is tried, a cesarean delivery becomes necessary. The safety of the mother and the baby is the prime consideration. Should a cesarean be necessary, you will be more comfortable and confident if you have previously discussed an alternative family-centered birth plan with your physician or midwife.

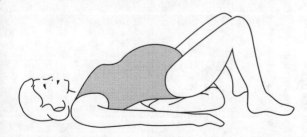

ROTATING A BREECH: There is a special exercise recommended by Dr. DeSa Sousa which she found to be 89% effective in her practice for rotating breech babies to a head-down position. There is no known risk to mother or baby, so the exercise is certainly worth a try if your baby remains in a breech position after the seventh month of pregnancy. Simply lie on your back with your knees bent and your pelvis elevated 9 to 12 inches. Do this twice a day, 10 minutes each time, with an empty stomach and bladder. Use pillows to achieve comfortable elevation of your pelvis. Although no studies have been done to confirm the effectiveness of this exercise, the little time you spend doing this exercise will be worthwhile if your baby is one that turns. (OB-GYN News)

Cesarean Birth

The most important thing to remember about a cesarean delivery is that it is the birth of a child and that in most cases it can be a joyful, family-centered experience. It is wise for all parents to prepare for cesarean birth and to discuss their options with the physician who would perform the surgery if that should become necessary.

In rare cases such as prolapse of the cord, fetal distress, or placenta abruptio (premature separation of the placenta from the wall of the uterus), an emergency cesarean must be performed. In these cases, the mother is usually put to sleep with general anesthesia, and the father or labor partner may not be allowed to be present at the birth of the baby. Although the couple may not be able to share the birth, there will be plenty of time later to bond with the baby. The most important consideration is, of course, the health of the baby and the mother.

Generally, there are signs late in pregnancy or during labor which indicate the possible need for a non-emergency cesarean delivery, and the physician and parents can plan for a family-centered birth. Some of these signs include breech or shoulder presentation, baby's head will not fit through mother's pelvis (CPD), placenta previa (low lying placenta completely or partially covering cervix), active genital Herpes infection, failed induction, or an active labor which does not progress after many hours.

Possible Options for Cesarean Parents in a Non-emergency Situation

- If appropriate, mother allowed to go into labor spontaneously rather than scheduling the cesarean. A period of labor is very beneficial to the baby.
- If appropriate, mother allowed to labor to determine if a vaginal birth is possible.
- Mother to be awake for the birth with regional anesthesia administered.
- Father or labor partner to be present at the birth.
- No preoperative sedatives for mother which might make her groggy or drowsy during birth.
- Incision on uterus to be transverse.
- Mother's hands to be free during the surgery to touch the baby as soon as possible after the birth.
- If mother and her labor partner desire, mirrors placed or the screen lowered just at the moment of birth.
- The father or labor partner to be able to hold the baby as soon as possible after the birth and to show the baby to the mother.

- The mother to decide with the anesthesiologist/nurse anesthetist whether or not she needs a sedative or analgesia immediately after the birth. These might make her groggy or drowsy in the recovery room.
- The father or labor partner to carry the baby to the nursery.
- Bonding and breastfeeding time with the baby in the recovery room before the regional anesthesia has worn off.
- Eye medication delayed to allow for bonding time.

Preoperative Procedures

- Urine specimen usually required.
- Blood tests, including typing and crossmatching for blood.
- Enema sometimes required.
- Clipping of some pubic hair may be necessary if the hair will interfere with the operation.
- IV started.
- Blood pressure cuff on arm.
- Cardiac monitor may be attached.
- Anesthesia administered–epidural, spinal, or general.
- Foley catheter inserted into bladder.
- Anesthesia screen placed in front of mom to create sterile field (also blocks view).
- Surgical scrub of abdomen.
- Drapes placed around surgical site.

The Surgery and Birth

- The baby is usually born within five to ten minutes after surgery has begun.
- If the mother is awake for the birth she may feel tugging sensations in the abdomen, pressure in the chest, or light shoulder pain during the surgery. She will hear the sounds of suctioning and will smell a "burning" scent as blood vessels are cauterized to stop bleeding. Reassurance from her partner and slow paced breathing will help reduce anxiety.
- It usually takes about 45 to 60 minutes to repair surgically or "close" the incision. The time passes more quickly if the baby and partner can remain in the delivery room with the mother.

Recovery Room Procedures
Usual stay is 1 to 2 hours

- In some areas, the epidural catheter will be left in place for about 24 hours to administer pain medication. If not, the mother may ask for additional medication just before the catheter is removed to ensure a comfortable hour or so in recovery with her baby.
- Most hospitals now allow both labor partner and baby to stay in the recovery room with the mother if she is awake and alert and so desires. This is often the ideal time to begin breastfeeding, as the regional anesthesia has probably not yet worn off. Do not worry if the baby does not seem interested in nursing at this time – some are not. Cuddling at the breast is still beneficial.
- The nurse will frequently check vital signs such as pulse, respiration, and blood pressure.
- The nurse will also check the dressing and may massage the uterus to make sure it is firmly contracted. The latter will be uncomfortable, so use your breathing techniques!
- The IV and Foley catheter are usually left in for about 24 hours. You will have a liquid diet for the first few meals after birth.

Recovery in the Hospital

- Ask for a cesarean roommate if at all possible.
- It is certainly possible and desirable to breastfeed following a cesarean birth. You will need extra pillows and extra help from the nurses to position the baby comfortably. Some mothers find it most comfortable to nurse while lying down; others find that a sitting position puts less strain on the incision.
- It is also desirable to have rooming-in. The father or partner can stay in the room with the mother the first day or two to help care for the baby. However, if you do not have someone to stay with you to help care for the baby and you decide to delay rooming-in until the second or third day when you are feeling stronger and more rested, do not feel guilty! If you are breastfeeding, have the nurses bring the baby in for demand feedings when you are not rooming-in in order to get your breastmilk supply well established.
- It is very important to move around as soon as possible. The sooner you can get up and walk, the speedier your recovery. Try to stand up straight and avoid the "cesarean shuffle" (leaning over to walk).
- You will have vaginal bleeding (lochia) just the same as if you delivered the baby vaginally.

- To minimize gas pains, avoid very hot, very cold, or carbonated beverages. Walking will help your body eliminate the gas. Begin the following abdominal exercise as soon as possible:

    Take a deep breath in, then slowly let out all the air, pulling in your abdominal muscles as you do so. Repeat 6 times each hour you are awake until you begin to pass gas.

- Even if you are breastfeeding, you can and should take pain medication if you are uncomfortable. Remind your doctor you are nursing so that he can prescribe the appropriate drug.
- For sore elbows, try using old socks with the toe cut out.
- Keep visitors to a minimum so that you can get plenty of rest.
- Ask your doctor to explain fully your surgery to you and to answer any questions you may have.
- If you were asleep for the delivery, ask the nurse who was there to tell you all about the birth of your baby.

Possible Emotional Feelings of Cesarean Parents

- Elation at the birth of their baby.
- Relief that it's finally over and baby is OK.
- Anger at not being able to have a vaginal delivery.
- Anger if the mother had to have general anesthesia and/or the father or labor partner could not be present at the birth.
- Estrangement from the baby if the mother was asleep or the father was not present at the birth.
- Disappointment if the birth experience did not meet expectations.
- Resentment at baby, father or labor partner, physician, or hospital staff.
- Guilt that mother did something to cause the cesarean.
- Worry about recovery period and scar.
- Fear about future pregnancies and the need for future cesareans.

Some couples experience only positive feelings with a cesarean, but most experience at least some of the negative feelings. Sometimes just talking them out with one another and knowing that other couples have felt the same feelings is enough. Other times, couples may find it helpful to talk with someone from a cesarean support group.

Recovery at Home

Don't try to be superwoman! You are recovering from major surgery as well as the birth of a baby. Plan to take it very easy for at least two weeks and plan to nap daily for at least six weeks. Your first priorities should be getting breastfeeding off to a good start and establishing new family bonds. Get help with the housework and cooking so that you can rest and spend your time with the baby.

- Keep necessary supplies such as diapers, pitcher of water, and nutritious snacks close by.

- Use a diaper service or disposable diapers.

- Use paper plates and cups.

- Check with your physician regarding recommendations for bathing. Most suggest no tub baths until the steri-strips have been removed.

- Your incision may itch for many months. Warm compresses and gentle scratching will help.

- Limit visitors.

- Drink plenty of liquids and eat a well balanced diet.

- Rest as needed.

- Discuss your feelings and postpartum adjustments with your husband and/or family members, and other cesarean mothers.

- Plan outings with or without the baby as soon as possible. A small pillow will cushion your incision from the seatbelt.

- Above all, relax and enjoy these first few weeks as a new family. It's incredible how quickly the time passes!

Vaginal Birth After Cesarean
VBAC – pronounced "vee-back"

A major change in maternity care in the recent years has been the shift from the old dictum "once a cesarean, always a cesarean" to the active encouragement of vaginal birth for mothers who have previously delivered by cesarean. The American College of Obstetricians and Gynecologists (ACOG) recommends that physicians identify women who are candidates for VBAC, counsel them regarding risks and benefits, and offer them a trial of labor. Studies have clearly shown that VBAC births are safer for both the mother and baby than repeat cesarean delivery. A vaginal birth presents less risk of infection, blood loss, urinary tract or bowel injury, and blood clots due to surgery. Recovery from vaginal birth is easier and faster than from surgery, so a mother may be more readily able to care for her newborn. In addition to the physical considerations, there are often significant psychological and financial benefits. For the baby, there is less risk of prematurity and breathing complications if labor begins spontaneously, rather than by scheduling a delivery date too soon.

ACOG estimates that between 60% and 80% of women who choose to labor can safely have a vaginal birth; the remainder will have another cesarean. The VBAC rate increased in the United States from 12.6% in 1988 to 28.3% in 1996. Gradually the rate decreased to 16.4% in 2001.

VBAC has proved successful so that it is no longer considered a "high-risk delivery." In many areas, VBACs are done in Birthing Rooms (or LDRPs) and are managed in exactly the same way as other "low-risk births." Women who would like to consider a vaginal birth after cesarean are encouraged to discuss this option with their doctor or midwife early in their pregnancies. A particularly good book on VBAC is *Birth After Cesarean: The Medical Facts* by Bruce Flamm, M.D.

Unexpected Outcomes

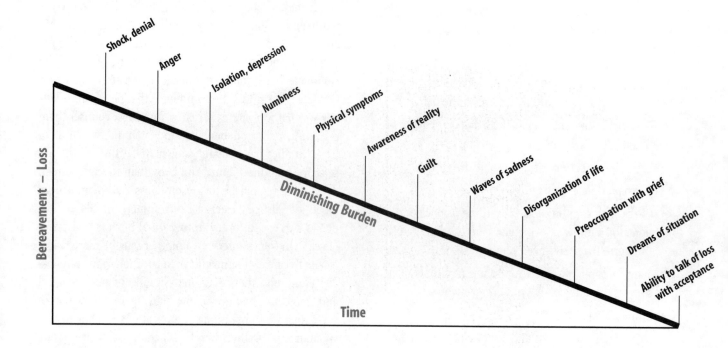

The Loss of a Dream

Regardless of the hopes and dreams we have about pregnancy and birth, there are no guarantees. For most, birth is a time of joy and relief, but sometimes when the unexpected occurs, it turns to a time of grief. Miscarriage or death of a newborn are obvious times of grief, but the cause for grief is not always death. Grief can be caused by a birth defect or injury, or even a birth experience that did not meet one's expectations. For some, a cesarean delivery is a cause for grieving, if that possibility had not been included in the birth plan. The needs of a couple and the psychological adjustments that must be made are the same, regardless of the cause for grief, however insignificant the problem may seem to others. The stations leading to acceptance of the loss as outlined above may be passed through in a matter of weeks, or may take many months. The time frame is rarely the same for all family members. Be patient with one another and realize that both anger and guilt are especially heavy burdens that can cause friction in a relationship. One may feel angry at the partner who already feels guilty, and this only magnifies the problem. Seek out others who have survived the problem that confronts you. Your nurse, health care provider, or childbirth educator may be able to put you in contact with an appropriate support group.

The Loss of a Baby

If a baby dies, most parents are better able to accept the loss if they have a chance to hold the baby and have pictures taken. Mementos such as a lock of hair, footprints, or an ID bracelet are helpful for parents to have for future memories. Naming the baby and holding a funeral or memorial service helps to bring the short life to closure. Final acceptance of a loss is hastened by an open discussion of feelings within the family or within a support group. Frequently there is another psychological upheaval on the anniversary date of the death.

It is good to have a basic understanding of the grieving process, as grief comes to us all at some point in our lives.

- Understand the normal stages of grief.

- Grieve in your own way and time.

- Cry to relieve pain and tension. It is healthy.

- Express your feelings to your partner and listen as your partner shares with you.

- Accept the fact that men and women may grieve in different ways.

- Locate a support group with others who have faced a problem such as you face.

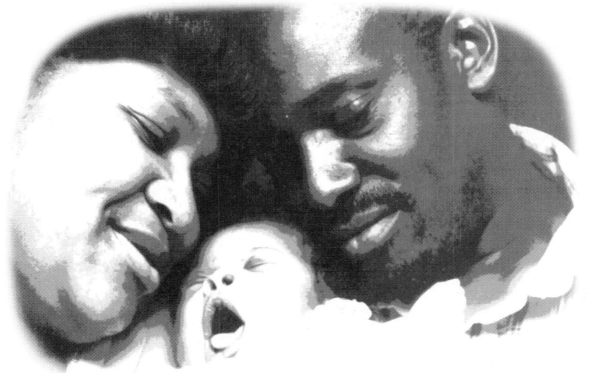

Postpartum and Family

People tell you how tired you'll be, but they don't tell you…that you'll be able to survive without much sleep because the simple act of looking at your baby is stirring, gratifying, energizing.

Carol Weston

The Postpartum Period

The first couple of hours after your baby's birth is sometimes called the fourth stage of labor. Your body is adjusting to its new, nonpregnant state. After the placenta has separated from the wall of the uterus, the uterus must contract firmly to prevent excessive bleeding (it will feel like a firm, grapefruit-sized mass at about the level of your navel). The nurse will massage your fundus (do slow paced breathing to decrease the discomfort), check the amount of vaginal flow (lochia), and monitor your pulse and blood pressure frequently until you have completed the recovery period (usually one to two hours). If you have had an episiotomy, an ice pack may be applied to reduce swelling.

Studies have shown that bonding is facilitated by early interaction between the new baby and his parents. You will be given an opportunity to touch and to hold your baby soon after birth. This can be a very special time to begin to get to know your infant, as most newborns are awake and alert for the first hour after birth. This is also a good time to initiate breastfeeding, since the baby will often suck or nuzzle the breast during this alert period.

Possible Physical Discomforts and Suggestions

Discomfort	Suggestions
Pain from repair of episiotomy	• Apply ice pack first 12 to 24 hours. • Take warm sitz baths or tub baths. • Kegel to promote circulation. • Apply topical anesthetics (sprays or foams). • Use "Tucks" (witch hazel compresses). • Request analgesics (remind your doctor if you are breastfeeding).
Inability to urinate	• Drink lots of liquids. • Run water in sink while you are trying to urinate. • Pour warm water over perineum as you are trying to urinate. • Do Kegel exercise.
Fear of having first bowel movement	• Talk with doctor or midwife about stool softener. • Drink lots of fluids. • Eat foods high in bulk – whole grains, bran, raw vegetables, fresh and dried fruits. • If no bowel movement, request suppository, laxative, or enema before leaving hospital.
Hemorrhoids	• Keep bowel movements as soft as possible. • Apply topical anesthetics. • Use "Tucks" (witch hazel compresses). • Kegel to promote circulation. • Discuss other medications with caregiver.
Afterbirth contractions *Normal to feel while breastfeeding* *More intense for multigravid mothers*	• Do slow paced breathing. • Use relaxation techniques—release all muscle groups. • Request analgesics.
Breast discomforts	• See page 63.

Possible Postpartum Problems

Most women are now home from the hospital or birth center within 12 to 48 hours after giving birth. Because your time in the hospital is so short, you may want to limit visitors so that you can use this time to gain experience in caring for your baby and get breastfeeding off to a good start.

This period is usually rather hectic, but before going home, take the time to ask your caregiver if there is any reason for you to limit activities such as driving, lifting, climbing stairs, sex, or exercise. This advice may vary, depending upon your physical condition and individual circumstances.

There is a certain amount of normal discomfort following birth (see chart on page 57), but some signals are important for you to be aware of in order to avoid more serious problems.

Call your Doctor or Midwife if:

* your vaginal discharge (lochia)
  – is excessive (filling one pad or more per hour)
  – turns bright red instead of dark red to brown
  – changes to foul smelling odor
  – contains blood clots larger than a golf ball
* you experience pain or cramping
  – in legs, arms, or chest
  – in abdomen
  – with urination
* your breast(s) develop
  – reddened areas or streaks
  – hot, tender, or painful lump(s)
* your abdominal incision
  – pain increases rather than decreases
  – develops drainage, or red streaks appear
  – begins to separate
* you are unable to have a bowel movement
* your breathing becomes difficult
* you develop a fever over 100.5°
* you experience blurred vision
* you have severe headaches
* you experience prolonged (beyond 2 weeks) "postpartum blues"

Possible Postpartum Emotions

If the possible physical discomforts following the birth of your child were an unhappy surprise to you, then the possible emotional feelings can provide even more of a challenge. Many women experience some degree of depression or "postpartum blues" following the birth of a child.

These "blues" are probably a combination of many factors including:

* Hormonal changes
* Physical discomforts
* Fatigue
* Letdown after looking forward to the birth for so long
* Disappointment at not immediately regaining your pre-pregnant shape
* Anxiety about assuming total responsibility for an infant
* Adjustment to the boredom and loneliness of staying home after working
* Worry about returning to work
* Balancing the needs of an infant with those of other family members

Sometimes it seems that there are not enough hours in the day to get everything done; while at the same time, it seems that there are too many hours left in the day until your husband comes home to provide some adult companionship and assume some of the responsibility for the baby. These "blue" feelings can last days for some women, weeks and even months for others. The most important thing to remember about this period is that it is normal to have negative and "blue" feelings from time to time and that it will get better. If depressed feelings persist or intensify; if you feel unable to properly care for your baby; or if you have thoughts of harming your baby; seek help from your health care provider immediately. Usually by 6 to 8 weeks postpartum, you will have regained your strength, the baby will have settled into some kind of schedule, and your family will have developed some new routines to accommodate the needs of the baby. Also at this time, the baby usually starts smiling and it all seems definitely worthwhile. To help you with those first trying weeks, however, here are some suggestions that have helped other new moms:

* Room-in at the hospital. Research has shown that mothers who room-in have fewer and/or shorter periods of baby blues.

* Let your emotions out! If you feel like crying, go ahead and cry. Share your feelings with your husband. He may be experiencing many of the same feelings.

* Be a supermom! But don't try to be Superwoman. Housework, social commitments, volunteer activities, and work-related activities should all take a backseat to becoming a mom. Take care of yourself as you recover, bond with your baby, get breastfeeding off to a good start, and enjoy your new family.

- Don't get dressed for the first week unless staying in your pajamas causes you to become depressed. If you are not dressed, you will be more likely to go back to bed when the baby naps and perhaps visitors will stay a shorter time.

- Plan to nap daily for the first six weeks, especially if you are nursing.

- Get help with the housework and cooking. If a friend asks what she can do to help, tell her to bring dinner. If you are planning to use cloth diapers, use a diaper service or disposable diapers for the first few weeks.

- Realize that almost all babies have their days and nights mixed up when they come home from the hospital and that almost all babies cry much more than you expected. It is all right to have occasional negative feelings and to wonder why you ever wanted to do this. Talking with friends who have young children or getting to know couples from your childbirth class can be comforting. It is helpful to know that others have experienced similar joys and frustrations.

For the New Father

With the birth of your child, you may experience a variety of strong emotions—pride, relief that your wife and child are fine, and a realization that lifelong responsibilities have begun.

Returning home to a new routine of diaper changes, sleepless nights, emotional ups and downs, well-meaning visitors, and a crying baby can be overwhelming. You may experience the "baby blues" with as much intensity as your wife does. While you are proud of your wife and fascinated with your new heir, you may grow impatient with meals from the freezer (or preparing your own), interrupted sleep, a less than tidy home, and having to share your wife's affection with your child. You want to offer emotional support to your wife, but you deserve emotional support as well. You may wonder why you ever wanted to become a father!

To ease this transition into fatherhood, it helps to become involved with the care of the baby right along with mom. Learning together and sharing feelings helps a couple understand one another's frustrations and joys. Just as you have shared the birth of your baby and gained a new appreciation for your wife, so now you will share in parenting your child. Although you have a new role as a parent, it is still important to remember your needs as a couple. Make time for each other. Love, understanding, and communication are essential. Being a parent is a lifelong team effort which produces many frustrations, but many more rewards.

Resuming Your Sexual Relationship

Like pregnancy, the postpartum period can be a very stressful time in a couple's sexual relationship. In fact, many couples wonder if sex will ever be like it was before the baby. A couple may be apprehensive that intercourse will be painful and possibly hurt the episiotomy site. A woman who is breastfeeding may find that her vaginal lubrication is inadequate and that penetration is indeed uncomfortable. The postpartum period is also a period of extreme fatigue for both parents, hardly conducive to romantic feelings. In addition, newborns are very emotionally demanding of their mothers and require much physical contact. Some women who share this intimacy with their infants throughout the day want a "breather" when the baby is finally in his crib in the evening. They may avoid physical contact with their husbands because they are emotionally drained by the baby's demands.

Bearing in mind all these negative factors, it is also true that this is one of the times in a couple's relationship when a satisfying sex life can most benefit their relationship. The postpartum woman often feels "fat" and unattractive and needs the assurance that her mate still finds her sexually attractive. Both parents need to know that their own intimate relationship and love for each other will not be changed by their new role as parents. Until both feel ready for intercourse, just kissing and cuddling can be a boost to a relationship.

Suggestions that other couples have found helpful:

- Set aside a special time for sexual relations when someone else has the baby or when the baby has just been fed and you are fairly certain he will sleep for a while. Take advantage of quiet mornings and afternoons when you both are well rested.

- You will ovulate and therefore may become pregnant before your first period returns. For information on family planning, consult your health care provider.

- Talk to each other – share your desires and your feelings!

What Pediatricians Are Saying About Breastfeeding

The American Academy of Pediatrics (AAP) has been a strong proponent of breastfeeding since 1948. However, based on recent scientific studies documenting the benefits of breastfeeding to the baby, the mother, the family, and to society, in 1997 the nation's pediatricians significantly strengthened their recommendations regarding breastfeeding:

"Human milk is the preferred feeding for all infants, including premature and sick newborns, with rare exceptions."

"Exclusive breastfeeding is ideal nutrition and sufficient to support optimal growth and development for the first 6 months after birth."

"It is recommended that breastfeeding continue for at least 12 months, and thereafter for as long as mutually desired."

In addition to the benefits of breastfeeding outlined in the following chart, breastfeeding has also been related to possible enhancement of the child's cognitive (brain) development. This positive relationship between breastfeeding and cognitive development was strengthened by the publication in the January 1998 journal, *Pediatrics*, of a study of more than 1000 children over an eighteen year period. Researchers in this study concluded that breastfeeding can positively influence childhood IQ scores and performance on standardized achievement tests throughout the school years.

Strong evidence exists that human milk reduces the incidence/severity of	A number of studies show a possible protective effect of human milk against	A number of studies indicate the following health benefits to the mother	Significant social and economic benefits to the nation include
Diarrhea Lower respiratory infection Ear infections (otitis media) Bacteria in the blood (bacteremia) Bacterial meningitis Botulism Urinary tract infection Severe inflammation of the intestines and colon (necrotizing enterocolitis)	Sudden infant death syndrome (SIDS) Insulin-dependent diabetes Ulcerative colitis Crohn's disease Cancer in the lymphatic system (lymphoma) Allergic diseases Other chronic digestive diseases	Less postpartum bleeding and more rapid return of the uterus to pre-pregnant size Earlier return to pre-pregnant weight Increased childspacing due to delayed resumption of ovulation (and menstruation) Less blood loss over the months following delivery due to lack of "periods" Reduced risk of premenopausal breast cancer Reduced risk of ovarian cancer Reduction in hip fractures in the postmenopausal period	Lower incidence of illness in the breastfed infant allows parents more time for siblings and other family duties, and reduces parents' absences from work and lost income At least $800 to $1200 savings in formula costs per baby during the first year Significant savings in health care costs due to fewer and shorter hospitalizations, fewer office visits, and decreased need for medications

Adapted from *AAP Policy Statement*, as reported in *Pediatrics*, Volume 100, December 1997.

In addition to the many health benefits, nursing can become a very convenient and natural bonding experience for mother and baby. However, sometimes the road to this wonderful experience is a little rocky. These are some hints that the American Academy of Pediatrics has given us to help smooth the way to get breastfeeding off to a good start:

- Breastfeeding should begin as soon as possible after birth, usually within the first hour.

- Newborns should be nursed when they show signs of hunger, such as increased alertness or activity, mouthing, or rooting. Crying is a late indicator of hunger.

- Newborns should actively nurse 10-15 minutes on each breast at each feeding.

- No supplements (sugar water, formula, etc.) should be given to breastfeeding newborns unless a medical indication exists.

- Supplements and pacifiers should be avoided whenever possible and, if used at all, only after breastfeeding is well established.

Remember that at the same time you are learning to breastfeed, you will be coping with other adaptations of the postpartum period: the mother's physical discomforts following childbirth, fatigue of both mother and father, and adjusting to the responsibility of caring for an infant 24 hours a day. Sometimes it seems easy to blame the baby's frequent crying and need for nighttime feedings on the lack of quality or quantity of mother's milk. In reality, most newborns, whether bottlefed or breastfed, cry 2 to 3 hours per day and get up during the night to eat!

You may feel encouraged that breastfeeding is going as it should, if you can answer yes to the checklist on page 100.

Support and Encouragement

Mothers who receive support and encouragement to continue nursing past these first hectic weeks most often find that nursing fulfills all their expectations. While you are still pregnant, select a knowledgeable support person whom you will call with questions or possible problems with nursing. This could be a sister or friend who has successfully breastfed her own child and is supportive of your breastfeeding, a La Leche League leader, lactation consultant, or your childbirth or breastfeeding educator. Learn as much as possible about breastfeeding. Knowledge of the process is key to building self-confidence.

Frequent Feedings in Early Weeks

The production of breastmilk is directly related to the frequency of nursing. Each time you put your baby to breast, a hormone is released in your body that stimulates your breasts to make more milk. Positioning your baby correctly and helping her to latch-on properly will assure that she nurses effectively. As milk is removed, more milk is made. Most newborn babies will nurse at least 8 to 12 times per 24 hour period, or about every 1½ to 3 hours. Later on, the baby may go longer between feedings, but in the first months, trying to put a baby on a strict schedule most often results in an inadequate milk supply. Giving supplemental formula during the first few weeks of life can interfere with this delicate supply-and-demand balance and cause the baby to nurse less frequently, thus decreasing the mother's milk supply.

Remember that all babies go through periodic growth spurts when they seem to nurse all the time. To meet his increased need, let the baby nurse more frequently. This is his way of increasing your milk supply. Try to get some extra rest, and be assured that growth spurts last only a few days.

Avoid Bottle Nipples, Pacifiers, and Nipple Shields

The sucking action of the baby's mouth on the breast is completely different from the sucking action on a bottle. Many orthodontists agree that the sucking of breastfeeding helps to develop the jaw more completely. If given even a few bottles in the early days of life, some babies may develop "nipple preference" or "nipple confusion," preferring a bottle nipple over the breast. They may refuse to take the breast, preferring the easy flow of milk from the bottle nipple. Tell the nurses that you intend to breastfeed exclusively in the early weeks and request that no bottles be given.

The American Academy of Pediatrics and many lactation consultants discourage the use of pacifiers for the healthy newborn, preferring that babies meet their sucking needs at the breast, at least until nursing is well-established.

Nipple shields are no longer recommended for sore nipples. The best remedy for sore nipples is improved positioning of the baby. He should take as much of the top and bottom of the areola in his mouth as possible, not just the nipple. It may be helpful to apply one of the following to the nipple and areola: warm, moist compresses; expressed breastmilk; or pure hospital-grade lanolin.

Breastfeeding Guide

	What's Happening	What to Expect	What You Can Do
Prenatally	The pregnancy hormones in your body are preparing your body for breastfeeding.	• Your breasts gradually become larger, firmer, and more tender. • The brown part around your nipple (areola) becomes larger, darker, and develops small bumps called Montgomery glands. These glands are thought to secrete an antiseptic lubricant that decreases dryness. • Colostrum, a thick yellowish liquid, may or may not leak from the breasts.	• Take a breastfeeding class. • Avoid using soap on the nipples, which may wash away the natural lubrication. • Determine if your nipples are everted, flat, or inverted. If flat or inverted, discuss strategies with your breastfeeding instructor or lactation consultant to aid early nursing. • It is not recommended that you try to hand-express colostrum.
Immediately After Birth	The delivery of the placenta causes a drop in estrogen and progesterone, which stimulates initial milk production.	The baby may be eager to nurse on one or both breasts immediately after birth, or he may not be interested at all. Even if he does not appear interested in nursing immediately, hold him skin-to-skin against your chest. Research indicates that spending time with your baby skin-to-skin helps him learn to breastfeed sooner.	• Nurse as soon as possible after birth to further stimulate milk production (early, frequent feeding may also help to prevent jaundice and engorgement). • Nurse at night even if not rooming-in. • Nurse on each side every 1½-3 hours as the baby desires. Wake the baby to feed during the day. • Learn different nursing positions. • In order to avoid "nipple confusion," avoid bottle nipples and pacifiers.
3-5 Days After Birth	Your milk will come in.	• Your breasts may feel very full and heavy. • They may become engorged—firm and uncomfortable. This early engorgement will disappear spontaneously. • Nipples feel the most tender at this time.	• If you are still in the hospital, continue rooming-in and frequent feedings. • If you are at home, continue to get plenty of rest. Continue short, frequent nursings. Wake the sleepy baby to feed 8 to 12 times every 24 hours. • If you are engorged, nurse frequently. • Take warm showers and hand-express to remove some of the milk. • Use cold compresses for comfort.
Ten Days After Birth	If you had engorgement, it usually has subsided. Normal swelling of your lymph glands has also decreased so that your breasts may actually feel smaller.	• Babies tend to be very fussy at about 10 days which may coincide with the disappearance of your engorgement; you may feel that you are not producing enough milk. This is usually not the case; just a coincidence. • Nipple soreness should be gone by 10-14 days.	• Lie down to nurse to increase rest. • Continue to take naps during the day when the baby sleeps. You still need extra rest! • Continue frequent nursings. Most newborns need at least 8 to 12 feedings every 24 hours. • Contact a lactation consultant if nipples are still sore at 10 to 14 days.
One Month After Birth	You are often resuming many activities you pursued before the pregnancy.	• The baby may experience a growth spurt, needing to nurse even more frequently for 24-48 hours in order to build up your milk supply. At this age babies still tend to be fussy for many reasons other than hunger.	• You still need extra rest during the day. • Share your feelings (both positive and negative) with your spouse and your friends. Do something special for you and your spouse or just for yourself. • Be assured that if your baby is only on breastmilk, 6 to 8 wet diapers per day indicates that he is getting plenty to eat! (Also, see page 100.)
Six Weeks After Birth	Hooray! Usually you are "feeling yourself" again and have recovered physically from the birth.	The baby, too, seems much happier. He is starting to coo and smile often. He seems to maintain some kind of pattern of feeding (although the pattern may change frequently).	• Keep up the good work! • Try to rest when you're tired. • Continue frequent nursings and *expect* some periodic growth spurts when the baby needs to nurse "all the time" in order to build up your supply of breastmilk. • Enjoy this very special time in your family's life.

Breastfeeding Challenges and Solutions

Challenge	Solution
Inverted or flat nipples	• During pregnancy, have your health care provider check to see if either of your nipples is inverted. (An inverted nipple, in response to cold, will retract rather than protrude.) • If your nipples are flat or inverted, discuss strategies with your breastfeeding instructor or lactation consultant to aid with early nursing. Frequent practice sessions with the baby before the milk comes in will help. Some lactation consultants may recommend breast shells, hard plastic cups with multiple ventilation holes which are worn inside the bra during the first weeks after the baby is born.
Engorgement	• Room-in and nurse frequently (every 1½-3 hours). • Wear a supportive bra for comfort. • Take a warm shower or apply warm compresses and hand express milk to soften areola before nursing. • Apply cold compresses between feedings.
Sore nipples	• Alternate nursing positions: sitting, lying down, or "football hold." • Make sure your positioning is correct. Baby should be tummy-to-tummy with mother. Both the baby's nose and the baby's chin should be touching the mother's breast. Support the breast during the feeding (see page 100). • Begin nursing on the least sore side first. • Massage breast to stimulate let-down reflex before putting baby to breast. • Make sure some of the lower portion of the areola is in the baby's mouth as well as the upper portion of the areola. • Use relaxation techniques and slow paced breathing when baby first begins sucking and for as long as necessary. • End feeding when baby is finished; do not allow the baby to sleep at the breast when nipples are sore. • Be sure to break suction before removing the baby from breast. • Air dry nipples after nursing. • Apply one of the following to the nipple and areola: warm, moist compresses; expressed breastmilk; or pure hospital-grade lanolin. • If using a breast pump, use the lowest setting that is effective. • Never use "bicycle-horn" type pumps or plastic bra liners.
Plugged ducts	• Apply warm compresses, or soak in warm tub before nursing. • Begin feeding on affected side. • Get baby's chin as close as possible to affected area. • Do breast massage while nursing. • Nurse twice on affected side during each feeding. • Try to eliminate causes such as too-tight bra.

Breastfeeding Challenges and Solutions

Challenge	Solution
Breast infection *Mastitis*	• Remove milk by continuing to nurse at frequent intervals, by hand expressing, or by using a breast pump. • Get baby's chin as close as possible to affected site. • Go to bed and rest. • Take antibiotics prescribed by your healthcare provider. • Apply warm compresses to affected breast.
Baby sleeping "too much"	• Newborns *do* need to nurse at least 8 to 12 times per 24 hour period. If your baby is not nursing at least this number of times, you will need to wake her every 2 to 3 hours during the day to nurse. Try the following to help wake up your baby: unwrap and undress her, change her diaper, talk to her, gently move her up and down and sideways, put her hand to her mouth, express a small amount of breast-milk so that she can smell it. It is usually not necessary to wake a baby at night to nurse unless she is not gaining weight adequately.
"Not enough milk"	• Although this is a common perception of new mothers, the truth is that most mothers make plenty of milk for their babies. Use the checklist on page 100 to determine whether or not breastfeeding is going well for you and your baby. • After evaluating the checklist on page 100, if you still feel that you may not be producing enough milk for your baby, contact either a nurse where your baby was born or a lactation consultant.

"Colicky" baby
Long periods of unexplained crying. Colic begins after the baby is two weeks of age and usually ends by 16 weeks.
	• Respond to early feeding cues before baby cries.
	• Continue to breastfeed frequently; changing to formula often makes symptoms worse.
	• The warmth and comfort of holding baby skin-to-skin while rocking, nursing, or sleeping may calm both of you.
	• A warm bath or warm compresses to the stomach may help.
	• Mother may try a change in her diet by eliminating one of the following, for one week at a time, to see if it helps:
	  – dairy products
	  – eggs
	  – nuts
	  – wheat

I'd like to breastfeed but I really want to lose weight quickly!

You may, in fact, lose weight more quickly as a breastfeeding mother than as a bottlefeeding mother, as production of milk consumes energy (calories). Strict dieting is not recommended for any new mother, whether breastfeeding or formula feeding, because of the physical and emotional recovery time necessary following childbirth. Breastfeeding mothers who combine healthy food choices with regular exercise most often experience the type of slow, gradual weight loss that is likely to be permanent.

Expressing Breastmilk

Many women who breastfeed today find that they need to express and store breastmilk. This can be done either by hand expression or with a breast pump. Because there are so many different types of pumps on the market, and because it is very important that the pump "fit" the mother properly, expert advice from a lactation consultant can be very useful.

An easy and inexpensive way to collect breast milk is by hand expression. To hand express, wash your hands with soap and water. Use both hands to massage your breast in a circular motion toward the nipple. Place your thumb and index finger on the areola (dark skin surrounding the nipple) about 1 to 1½ inches back from the nipple and press inward toward the chest wall, gently rolling the thumb and finger forward. Repeat until the milk stops coming; then change to a new location around the areola.

Many nursing mothers use hand expression or one of the cylinder hand pumps for occasional pumping. Bicycle-horn type hand pumps are not recommended because of their tendency to collect bacteria and cause excessive stress to the nipples.

Many small, battery-operated hand pumps require the mother to interrupt the vacuum periodically to create a suck-release cycle. Some models have settings which allow for the intensity of the vacuum to be adjusted, but many do not. Unless properly used, these pumps can cause nipple irritation. If purchasing a small battery-operated or electric hand pump, choose one with automatic cycling.

For mothers who pump on a regular basis, a hospital-grade, automatic electric pump is recommended. In addition to offering automatic suction and control of the vacuum, these pumps can be used with a double kit so that both breasts can be pumped at the same time. "Double-pumping" saves time and increases milk production. These pumps are available for rent throughout the nation for a reasonable cost and are also available for purchase. For information on these pumps, contact your childbirth educator or lactation consultant.

Before expressing milk by any method, wash your hands, then use both hands to massage the breast in a circular motion toward the nipple. This will stimulate the letdown reflex and encourage milk flow.

Storing and Freezing Breastmilk

- *Refrigeration.* According to the The American Academy of Pediatrics, you can store expressed breastmilk for your healthy newborn in a refrigerastor for up to 72 hours. Other researchers believe that expressed milk is safe in a refreigerator for about five days. If your baby is preterm or ill, it is recommended that you store breastmilk in the refrigerator for no more than 48 hours. It is a good idea to place the milk in the refrigerator soon after collecting. Place the milk in the back of the refrigerator where it is colder, rather than in the door.

- *Containers.* In order to preserve the infection-fighting properties of the milk, the best kind of container for storage is a glass or hard plastic bottle. Opaque containers protect the milk from sunlight, which may alter components in the breastmilk. The greatest loss of infection-fighting properties of breastmilk occurs with disposable plastic bags. This may not be a concern if the baby is taking a majority of her feedings directly from the breast. Glass or hard plastic bottles should be washed with hot, soapy water, and air dried after each use or washed and dried in a dishwasher.

- *Freezing.* If you have a standard home freezer that freezes to 0 degrees Fahrenheit, breastmilk can be frozen for up to 6 months. If you have a standard combination refrigerator-freezer with a separate door for the freezer, breastmilk can be frozen for up to 3 months. Always label the milk with the dates collected and use the oldest milk first. If you are collecting milk for a healthy newborn, you can collect a little milk each day and add it to the bottle or bag so it is frozen in layers. Before adding new milk to already frozen milk, chill the new milk in the refrigerator for several hours so that it will not thaw the already frozen breastmilk. For the preterm or ill baby, it is recommended that you store or freeze each collection of milk separately.

- *Thawing.* To thaw the frozen milk, hold the bottle or bag under cold running water, then under lukewarm running water. Never use a microwave or stove to thaw or heat breastmilk. Thawed breastmilk should be used within 24 hours. Always discard any remaining thawed breastmilk that the baby does not take. Do not refreeze.

Observations of a Pediatrician

During the nine months or so in which a woman is pregnant, she may develop a personal relationship with her unborn baby. She may call it by a pet name and even attribute to it certain personality characteristics. When the baby is born, there is sometimes the feeling of recognition of someone she has known for some time.

Dad, on the other hand, may greet the "little stranger" with much less sense of recognition. In fact, it may be several weeks before the infant is felt by dad to be a real individual, with a personality uniquely its own.

If the parents are expecting a smiling "bundle of joy," they may be in for a surprise when they see baby covered with a mixture of vernix caseosa, amniotic fluid, and occasionally blood or meconium. Until the baby breathes or cries, its skin may be more dusky blue or purple than it is white, brown, or black. For the unprepared parent, this may cause unnecessary concern, until the baby breathes and oxygen turns the skin a more normal color. Even then, the hands and feet of the normal infant may continue to have a bluish cast for some time. Molding of the head, allowing passage down the birth canal, is another normal feature which may cause parents anxiety. The baby's head returns to its normal shape within a few days.

Babies when first born must be kept warm to conserve body heat. After all, they are coming rather abruptly from an environment which has provided nourishment, waste disposal, protection from bumps, and a finely controlled temperature. So when the birth attendant bundles mom and baby together or places the baby in an infant warmer, it is to allow gradual adjustment of the body temperature to the extrauterine environment.

Within a few days after birth, many babies turn a yellow color. You may have heard of it as "jaundice," a term which means yellow. This is often perfectly natural—so-called physiologic jaundice. However, it may also indicate a problem, so you should check with your doctor to be certain. A blood test for bilirubin may be required to make the distinction. If the results are elevated, your doctor may recommend phototherapy to be performed at the hospital or at home.

For most babies, the best food is human breastmilk. Breastmilk may be expressed from the breast and frozen for later feeding; this is one way to allow dad to have some of the satisfaction of feeding the baby from time to time and will allow mom a needed several hours of uninterrupted sleep, or a night out. Families with a strong history of allergies should discuss the risks of formula with the baby's doctor before using it.

Many questions arise, even among knowledgeable parents of healthy, normal babies. Queries may relate to the "soft spot" on the baby's head (it's normal, and needs no special protection), to the baby's umbilical cord (keep it clean and dry to avoid infection), to the bowel movements (they may occur several times a day, whenever the baby eats, or they may be several days apart in the older infant, and still be normal), to circumcision (there are reasons not to do it, and reasons to do it; you should talk it over with your doctor). Don't hesitate to bring any issue up for discussion, whether your concerns arise either before or after your baby is born.

Don't push the panic button...but it's time to call your doctor

...when your baby, who has been feeding well, loses interest in eating for a couple of feedings in a row;

...when your baby fails to gain weight;

...when the area around the umbilicus looks red, swollen, and angry;

...when there is blood or mucus in the bowel movements;

...when the baby is lethargic, or does not move about, even though awake;

...if the baby becomes jaundiced;

...when the baby feels either too hot or too cool to the touch, despite a normal room temperature and appropriate clothing or coverings; or,

...when either mom or dad are concerned that something may be wrong with the baby's health.

Gordon Green, M.D.

Life With Baby

Sleeping, Crying, and Consoling

Most babies will sleep less or cry more than new parents expect. The *average* newborn sleeps 13 to 17 hours a day, and may cry for one to four hours a day. (That means a new baby may cry up to half his waking hours, and be normal!) The *very quiet* or *very active* infant will sleep or cry less than or more than the *average* baby. Crying is the only way a baby has to communicate. This new language may be frustrating to you as you learn to translate it. Your baby may cry to signal a physical need of hunger, fatigue, pain, or of discomfort such as needing a diaper changed or being too hot or too cold. Or crying may indicate an emotional need to be held and to be sociable. A baby may cry when he is lonely or bored or when he has had too much stimulation and play. As you get to know your baby, you will more easily distinguish the sudden piercing cry of pain, the whiny continuous cry of fatigue, and the stop-and-start cry of hunger. If he stops crying when you pick him up, it may be that he was just lonely or bored. Most experts today believe that it is important to respond to your baby's cry and try to meet both his physical and emotional needs. A baby's first task is to learn to trust. By answering his cries, you are helping him establish trust with the world. You won't spoil him by meeting his needs for cuddling and socializing; rather you are teaching him respect and security.

Temperament

Like each labor and birth experience, each baby is unique. Even in the womb, one mother may note that her baby moves about vigorously at any hour of the day or night, while another mother relates more gentle movements according to a regular pattern. Some babies have calm, passive dispositions and are quiet much of the time. When awake they may lie peacefully, pacifying themselves and moving with slow, smooth movements. Some have such a quiet intensity about them that they may even appear to be depressed. Other babies are extremely demanding and want to be held and rocked seemingly all the time. Their movements are thrusting and vigorous, and their cries are long and loud. Yet others who want constant attention are bubbly and happy when they get it. At first, a quiet baby may be perceived as unresponsive or an active baby as uncontrollable, but you will soon learn to understand and accept the temperament and activity of your child as normal for him or her.

It is wise to listen politely to the advice of friends and family, then to trust your own instincts of how to care for *your* child. What worked for others may or may not work for you. It is our own inborn temperaments that contribute to the dynamics within a new family.

Quiet Baby	Average	Active Baby
Cries rarely		. . . . .Cries frequently, loud and long
Sleeps much of the time		. . . . .Sleeps in short periods
Lies quietly, wide-eyed		. . . . .Wants attention when awake
Moves gently and slowly		. . . . .Moves with vigorous thrusts and kicks
Mouths and sucks fists gently		. . . . .Sucks vigorously
Enjoys bath, changing diapers		. .Cries and kicks through baths and diaper changes
Responds positively to holding, gentle rocking		. . . . . .Responds to vigorous pats, rocking, bouncing
Protests very little		. . . . .Protests often
Distracted from feeding by noise or object		. . . . .Nurses vigorously through distractions

Chart adapted from *Infants and Mothers* by T. Berry Brazelton, MD

States of Activity

Immediately after birth and for about ten percent of the time during the first week of life, most babies are in the **quiet alert state**—a time when you will see your baby's natural curiosity. Although their bodies are quiet, their eyes seek out human faces and they respond to the familiar voices of their parents.

After a short period in the quiet alert state, most babies will begin to move their arms and legs and enter into the **active alert state** — a time when baby is easily distracted and less able to focus his attention totally on you. This state precedes crying or drowsiness. You may be able to calm him, and head off the **crying state**, by putting him in a front pack or sling. Babies are often soothed by the warmth of being close to you, the sound of your heartbeat, and the movement as you walk. Slings or packs allow mom or dad to do some housework or shopping with hands free and baby happy. When old enough to control their heads well, many babies will enjoy a backpack.

Remember, while some babies are content being carried for hours, others need frequent changes of activity. A rocking chair or an infant swing may calm a fussy baby. All babies have a need to suck, but the use of pacifiers is discouraged for the newborn, until nursing is well established. After a few weeks, if you are certain that your baby is well nourished, and if he mouths his fist or makes sucking motions and seems discontent between feedings, he may be soothed with a pacifier.

The swing, the pack, rocking, or feeding a baby may make him **drowsy**, then he will fall asleep. Most babies alternate between **quiet sleep** and **active sleep** about every thirty minutes. Some babies will nurse well if they are picked up as they begin to awaken from active sleep and fed while still calm. Others need to fully awaken and express their desire to feed so they don't return to a sleep state before they have had enough to eat. You will soon learn which is better for your baby. When he returns to the quiet alert state, take advantage of the opportunity to play with your baby.

Playing With Your Newborn

Hold and talk to your baby face to face. Let him see you, smell you, feel your warmth, and hear your voice. These first interactions are important for you and your newborn. Babies often react to high pitched sounds before the lower pitches. During the first month, try the following "games."

- Talk or read, varying the pitch of your voice.
- Sing. (Babies don't care if you sing on key!)
- Exaggerate your facial expressions. Smile, frown.
- Stick your tongue out and in slowly and see if baby repeats your action.
- Stroke, massage your baby with gentle pressure from chest to fingers; chest to toes; head to toes.
- Straighten, then bend baby's arms at the elbow, legs at the knee, slowly and gently.
- Let baby grasp your thumbs while lying on his back. Gently help him stretch his arms over his head, then down by his side. At first, do arms together, then alternate with one arm up while other is down.
- Gently pump baby's legs, as riding a bicycle.
- Guide baby's hands to touch your face.
- Kiss and blow on baby's hands, feet, tummy.
- Shake a rattle, bell, keys, or a brightly colored ball about a foot from baby's face to let him "track" or follow the shape and sound as you slowly move it.
- As you carry your baby, describe the smells, sights, and sounds that you encounter.
- Look in a mirror together. Point to Mama, Daddy, Baby (using baby's name).
- Talk to your baby as you bathe him, change his diapers, dress him. Name the objects you use and tell him what you are doing.
- Play music and dance with your baby.

As your baby grows and experiences the world, you will see more positive rewards for your efforts. Take time to play!

Quiet Alert	Active Alert	Crying
Little to no movement	Frequent episodes of movement	Vigorous movement
Watch and listen attentively	Make small sounds	Communicate need
Eyes wide open and bright	Eyes open looking around	Eyes open or tightly closed

Drowsiness	Active Sleep	Quiet Sleep
Small movements; smiles, frowns, sucks	Slight movements; smiles, frowns, sucks	Body still
Waking or falling asleep	Breaths irregular and faster	Breaths regular
Eyes dull; no focus; eyes may roll upward	Eyes may flutter or move under lids	Eyelids closed and still

States of consciousness as described by Marshall and Phyllis Klaus in *The Amazing Newborn*

Ideas for Preparing Siblings

- Read books about new babies and encourage discussion about what new babies are like and what changes might occur within the family. Also, if the child seems interested, use books and discussions to answer questions about "where babies come from."

- Get out the older child's baby book and go through it with him, paying particular attention to how you cared for him when he was a young baby (a lot of time rocking, holding, nursing, etc.).

- If possible, borrow a young baby for a day to demonstrate baby care and let the older child participate in that care as much as possible.

- If you are planning a school, room, or bed change for the older child, do it as early in your pregnancy as possible so the older child doesn't feel "kicked out" by the baby.

- Encourage the older child to participate in getting things ready for the baby.

- If the child is mature enough, let him accompany you to the doctor and let him listen to the baby's heartbeat with a doppler or fetoscope. Look at books on fetal development together to trace the growth of the baby.

- Begin preparing the older child for the separation when mom will be in the hospital or birth center. Show the older child where mom will be. If he will be spending the night away from home, you might let him have a practice run.

- Enroll your child in a sibling preparation class.

- Record bedtime stories on cassette tapes that can be played while you are in the hospital or birth center. Say "good night" to your child at the end of the tape.

- Pack a new T-shirt that says "I'm a big brother (or sister)" and leave it with whoever is keeping your older child so they can give it to him as soon as the new baby is born.

- Call your older child as soon as the new baby arrives to tell him the good news (unless it's during the night). Don't be disappointed if he is not quite as excited as you are – it takes time!

- When you come home from the hospital, let daddy carry the baby so your arms are open for your older child.

- Let the older child hold and participate in the care of the baby as much as possible.

- Ask visiting friends and relatives to greet the older child and pay attention to him before greeting the baby.

- Read a story to the older child while feeding the baby.

- Try to plan a special time each day for just you and the older child.

- Expect some "acting out" or regressive behavior from the older child. After all, his adjustment to the new baby is at least as great as your adjustment to your first baby. What is really needed is lots of love and the reassurance that the new baby is not taking his place.

Recommended Reading List to Prepare Siblings

Alexander, Martha. *Nobody Asked Me If I Wanted a Baby Sister.*

Carroll, Teresa. *Mommy Breastfeeds Our Baby.* (La Leche League)

Cole, Joanna. *How You Were Born.*

Collman, Barbara J. *Kid's Book to Welcome A New Baby.* (activity book)

Corey, Dorothy. *Will There Be a Lap for Me?*

Gordon, Sol and Judith Gordon. *Did the Sun Shine Before You Were Born?* (facts of life)

Hoban, Russell. *A Baby Sister for Frances.*

Lansky, Vicki. *A New Baby at Koko Bear's House.*

Lindgren, Astrid. *I Want a Brother or Sister.* (La Leche League)

Mayle, Peter. *Where Did I Come From?*

Nilsson, Lennart. *How Was I Born?*

Pearse, Patrica and Edwina Riddell. *See How You Grow.* (facts of life)

Rogers, Fred. *The New Baby.*

Scott, Ann Herbert. *On Mother's Lap.*

Smith, Dian G. *My New Baby and Me.* (activity and record book)

Weiss, Joan Soloman. *Your Second Child.*

Recommended Resource List for Pregnant Couples

Pregnancy

American College of Obstetricians and Gynecologists. 2000. *Planning Your Pregnancy and Birth.*

Jiménez, Sherry. 1992. *The Pregnant Woman's Comfort Guide.*

Kitzinger, Sheila. 1996. *The Complete Book of Pregnancy and Childbirth.*

Nathanielsz, Peter & Christopher Vaughan. 2001. *The Prenatal Prescription.*

Nilsson, Lennart. 1986. *A Child is Born.*

Simkin, Penny, Janet Whalley, & Ann Keppler. 2001. *Pregnancy, Childbirth and the Newborn.*

Vaughan, Christopher. 1996. *How Life Begins – The Science of the Womb.*

Childbirth

Balaskas, Janet. 1992. *Active Birth.*

England, Pam & Rob Horowitz. 1998. *Birthing from Within.*

Giglio, Ann-Marie. 1999. *Labor Day: Shared Experiences from the Delivery Room.*

Goer, Henci. 1999. *The Thinking Women's Guide to a Better Birth.*

Harper, Barbara. 1994. *Gentle Birth Choices.*

Kitzinger, Sheila. 2001. *Rediscovering Birth*

Korte, Diana and Roberta Scaer. 1992. *A Good Birth, A Safe Birth.*

Lieberman, Adrienne. 1992. *Easing Labor Pain.*

Simkin, Penny. 2001. *The Birth Partner.*

Taylor, Catherine. 2002. *Giving Birth: A Journey Into the World of Mothers and Midwives*

Multiples

Gromada, Karen. 1999. *Mothering Multiples – Breastfeeding and Caring for Twins.*

Noble, Elizabeth. 1991. *Having Twins*

Luke, Barbara & Tamara Eberlein. 1999. *When You're Expecting Twins, Triplets, or Quads.*

Nutrition

Swinney, Bridget & Tracey Anderson. 2000. *Eating Expectantly.*

Exercise

Balaskas, Janet. 1999. *Easy Exercises for Pregnancy.*

Clapp, James. 2002. *Exercising Through Your Pregnancy.*

Noble, Elizabeth. 1995. *Essential Exercises for the Childbearing Year.*

Tupler, Julie. 1996. *Maternal Fitness.*

Breastfeeding

Eiger, Marvin, & Sally Olds. 1999. *The Complete Book of Breastfeeding.*

Huggins, Kathleen. 1999. *The Nursing Mother's Companion.*

La Leche League. 1997. *The Womanly Art of Breastfeeding.*

Newman, Jack & Teresa Pitman. 2000. *The Ultimate Breastfeeding Book of Answers.*

Pryor, Gale. 1997. *Nursing Mother, Working Mother.*

Pryor, Karen. 1991. *Nursing Your Baby.*

Renfrew, Mary, Chloe Fisher, & Suzanne Arms. 2000. *Bestfeeding: Getting Breastfeeding Right for You.*

Tamaro, Janet. 1998. *So that's what they're for!*

| Postpartum | Bing, Elisabeth & Libby Colman. 1997. *Laughter and Tears – The Emotional Life of New Mothers.* |
| | Placksin, Sally. 2000. *Mothering the New Mother – Your Postpartum Resource Companion.* |

Newborn Care	Brazelton, T. Berry. 1994. *Infants and Mothers.*
	Caplan, Frank, ed. 1995. *The First Twelve Months of Life.*
	Jones, Sandy. 1992. *Crying Baby, Sleepless Nights.*
	Klaus, Marshall and Phyllis Klaus. 2000. *Your Amazing Newborn.*
	Leach, Penelope. 1997. *Your Baby and Child: From Birth to Age Five*
	Neifert, Marianne, Nancy Dana, & Anne Price. 1993. *Dr. Mom – A Guide to Baby and Child Care.*
	Sears, William & Martha Sears. 2003. *The Baby Book: Everything You Need to Know About Your Baby from Birth to Age Two* .
	Sears, William. 1996. *The Fussy Baby Book.*

| Parenting | Clarke, Jean Illsley. 1998. *Growing Up Again.* |
| | Faber, Adele & Elaine Mazlish. 1999. *How to Talk So Kids Will Listen and Listen So Kids Will Talk.* |

Cesarean Birth and Vaginal Birth After Cesarean (VBAC)	Flamm, Bruce. 1992. *Birth After Cesarean: The Medical Facts.*
	Korte, Diana. 1998. *The VBAC Companion*
	Young, Diony, and Charles Mahan. 1989. *Unnecessary Cesareans – Ways to Avoid Them.* (ICEA)

| Doulas, Labor Support | Klaus, Marshall, Phyllis Klaus, and John Kennell. 2002. *The Doula Book.* |

Sources for Books and Information

Local libraries or bookstores are often an excellent source for childbirth related reading materials. You may also wish to contact the organizations listed below to obtain their listings of books, videotapes, or other information via phone, mail or the internet.

Lamaze International
Childbirth educator referrals and training
2025 M Street NW, Suite 800
Washington, DC 20036-3309
(800) 368-4404 or (202) 367-1128
Lamaze Bookstore (877) 952-6293
http://www.lamaze.org

ICEA *(International Childbirth Education Association)*
Childbirth educator referrals and training
P.O. Box 20048
Minneapolis, MN 55420
(612) 854-8660
ICEA Bookstore (800) 624-4934
http://www.icea.org

La Leche League
Referrals to breastfeeding support groups
Books and other Resources
P.O. Box 4079
Schaumburg, IL 60168-4079
(708) 519-7730
http://www.lalecheleague.org

DONA *(Doulas of North America)*
Doula referrals and training information
DONA central office
PO Box 626
Jasper, IN 47547
(888) 788-DONA
http://www.dona.org

Additional shopping via the Internet: Amazon Books at http://www.amazon.com

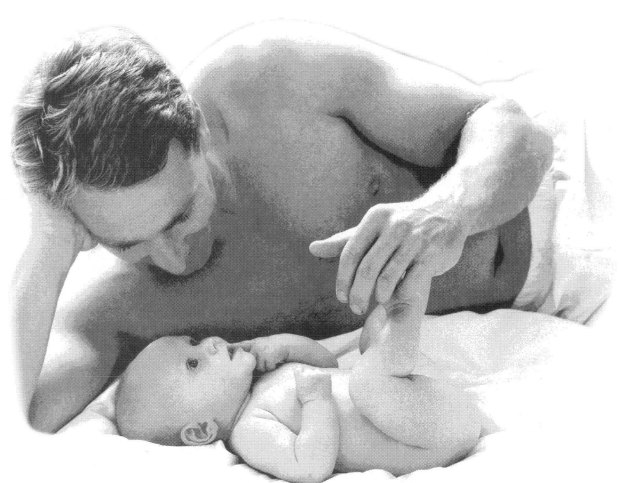

Birth Reports

The birth of a baby is an everyday miracle...a deep
and permanent memory for the birthing woman and
those who love her and support her.

Penny Simkin
The Birth Partner

Our Son Jeff

Giving birth to our son Jeff was one of the most exciting, miraculous, wonderful experiences of my life. With time I find I have forgotten many of the small details about the labor and birth, but the incredulous and awesome feeling of giving birth is still vivid in my mind.

The pregnancy went smoothly but turned out to be a long one. My due date of May 5th came and passed, the doctor said perhaps we miscalculated a bit and May 30 was more likely the date. Finally, on June 14, I went to the hospital for an oxytocin challenge test to determine if the placenta was still functioning properly since I was overdue. Pitocin was administered during the OCT test, and this eventually triggered a normal labor after I returned home from the test that afternoon. I stayed at home during most of the early and middle stages of labor just because I was more comfortable there than in the hospital. My contractions stayed about 5 minutes apart all afternoon and evening and were fairly strong but manageable. They seemed easy in contrast to the pitocin-induced contractions I had experienced during the 3-hour OCT test in the hospital that morning. The pitocin contractions came one right on top of another with no rest in between and it was extremely difficult for me to stay in control. I was better able to handle the contractions of natural labor that afternoon and evening because I had a couple of minutes or more in between contractions to rest and regroup. By this point in labor, I was very glad we had faithfully practiced all the techniques we learned in childbirth classes.

We finally went to the hospital about 10:30 that evening when the contractions began getting closer, about 3 minutes apart. Transition lasted about 45 minutes and was difficult, but my husband and the nurses kept telling me it was almost over and that kept me going. The pushing only took about 15 minutes. Jeff was born so quickly I could hardly believe it! When the doctor handed him to me, I was amazed at how alert Jeff was. He looked directly into my eyes as if to say, "Well, here I am!" and I was totally overwhelmed by the entire birth and life process.

No one could ever have totally prepared or described to us what a wonderful, joyful experience this birth would be. It is a moment in both our lives we will cherish always.

Sue Graham

From the moment my wife received word confirming that we were pregnant, we went from all the excitement of telling family and friends to being scared of the responsibilities and changes we would face.

As the months passed and the baby grew, my wife and he developed strong physical and emotional bonds. I had the feeling of being left out. I could feel the baby move, listen to sounds he made, but I was still an outsider. So for nine months, I stood by watching a relationship building without me.

Around the seventh month, my wife and I enrolled in a childbirth class. My wife decided she would like to try to have a non-medicated delivery, and that I would be participating as her labor partner. As her husband, I was 100% behind her, as an expectant father I had my doubts. I am not the type of person who copes well with loved ones who are in pain. But when my wife and I walked into the hospital that night, all those fears weren't there. I was too busy participating in the birth of our son.

In the delivery room, one of the most wonderful things in my life happened. I watched our baby being born. From the moment I saw his head crown, to when I saw his tiny head and face, then finally seeing the entire body of our healthy son, to telling my wife that we had a boy, it was incredible. I held Jeff in my arms for the first time and tears came to my eyes. Words can't tell of the happiness and joy I felt. These are moments I will remember forever.

Steve Graham

Cary's Birth Story

After waiting 32 years to have a baby, I was extremely excited when I found out I was pregnant, and a little "over eager" to soak up any information I could find on childbirth. So much so, that at 10 weeks, my husband Steve and I attended an early pregnancy class. Most everyone in the class was planning for an epidural, but I was curious about the possibility of natural childbirth. Our instructor suggested that we consider a doula; a concept we were not familiar with but one we were both very interested in.

My pregnancy was healthy and uneventful until the 30th week when we ended up with a midnight trip to the hospital with painful contractions. After discovering that the contractions were coming regularly every two minutes, I was given medication to help them stop, then sent home for 10 weeks of bedrest. This was a complete shock to us since pregnancy had gone so smoothly, but we followed our orders strictly in order to avoid a premature birth. The 10 weeks seemed to drag on with nothing to do but to read about, think about, and talk about the upcoming event and baby we so eagerly awaited. One helpful thing I did during this time was to watch the video of my sister's birth. Seeing her come through it so well, I was confident that I should be able to succeed too.

After a routine checkup at 37 weeks, my doctor was concerned that the baby might be very large and began talking about the possibility of inducing. I was not eager to do this, but at 38 weeks when he suggested using prostaglandin gel to soften my cervix, I agreed. The only effects I felt from the gel were slight cramps and the discomfort of having it inserted. At 41 weeks, and still no sign of labor, I was feeling extremely anxious and agreed to try the gel again that evening. At 6:00 the next morning, my water broke.

We arrived at the hospital at 7:30 after calling my doctor, my doula, our family, and a few friends. We had decided earlier that we wanted our family at the hospital, but the only people we planned to have in the birthing room were ourselves and our doula. At around 8:00, my doula arrived and I immediately felt calm. Her presence alone gave me a huge dose of confidence. Shortly after, I was seen by the doctor and told that if I wasn't in a regular labor pattern by noon, he wanted to induce. That was all the motivation I needed to take to the halls and walk. Steve was extremely nervous at this point and our doula sensed it and gave him some needed "time off." So I walked and walked and walked accompanied by Jeanne, stopping only to breathe through my contractions. The time spent walk-

ing and talking with her was very helpful in passing the time. Her gentle encouragement continued to boost my confidence making me think, "I can do this - I'm DOING this!" Up to this point, the contractions were only a little stronger than very hard menstrual cramps, but as noon approached, they started getting much more intense. It was around this time that my mother and sister arrived at the hospital. I hadn't expected to be so glad to see them or to be so overwhelmed with emotion when they entered the room. But when they came in, I knew that I wanted them to stay. The combination of doula, family, and spouse was perfect for me. I felt so loved and supported at all times – something I hadn't anticipated cherishing so dearly about the birth process.

I had progressed in dilation from barely a 1 to a 4 during this time. The time between noon and 3:00 was a blur of one strong contraction after another. The pain never felt too intense to handle, but I worked hard on remaining very focused on my breathing. Another helpful tool for me was music. I had tried out several relaxing CD's prior to labor and found one I was particularly fond of. I played it continuously throughout labor on my "walkman" which seemed to help me go deep inside myself during the particularly difficult contractions. I began to experience back labor and leg pain during this time and found much comfort in massage and touch that my sister and doula so freely gave.

At 3:00, I had progressed to an 8 and began feeling the urge to push, which for me was BY FAR the most difficult part of the labor process. In describing it to Steve, I said that it felt like a freight train was running through my body at full speed and I was having to hold it in. I began to have my first panicky feelings of doubt as this phase of labor wore on. If not for the continuous encouragement and sometimes rather specific instructions to "blow!," I would have fallen apart. At around 4:45 I was given the go ahead to push and I was determined that things were going to quickly "come to a head." I pushed with every ounce of strength I had whenever I felt the urge and within 4-5 pushes, Caroline's head was crowning. The doctor was not yet in the room and everyone was surprised when on the very next push, Caroline's entire head was out. Everything and everyone seemed to be moving in slow motion. I remember the nurse yelling for the doctor while telling me not to push, but all I cared about and all I could focus on was Caroline, the little head I saw in the mirror. I was oblivious to all else. The doctor did arrive and after another push, I had a beautiful (and average-sized) baby girl laying on my chest at 5:09 p.m. I had a small tear that required a few stitches, but I wasn't phased by it after laying eyes on Caroline. She was extremely alert for several hours and my sister remarked that she seemed like an old soul – very wise, the way she gazed so intently at each of us. After the birth, I felt completely exhilarated and euphoric. I felt invincible and capable of accomplishing anything. I hadn't known fully what to expect from a natural childbirth, but it far surpassed my highest expectations and wildest dreams, and I would never want to do it any other way. These wonderful feelings came in handy and helped me not to become too discouraged when we had difficulty breastfeeding.

Caroline didn't seem interested in breastfeeding and had difficulty latching on from the very beginning. I was nervous and unsure and hearing her shriek and arch away from me when I put her to my breast was very disheartening. I was prepared through my reading and childbirth classes that it didn't always happen perfectly right away so I wasn't completely discouraged. But it was unsettling and it began to eat away at my confidence. I felt labeled as "the one who cannot nurse" and began to feel truly discouraged when they wanted me to give her formula. My mother and sister kept encouraging me to stick with it which helped tremendously.

Our nursing problems continued for 2 weeks. The only way I could get her to take any breastmilk was to pump and feed her from a bottle. I would continue to offer her my breast and she continued to reject it. I had all but given up hope and resolved to pump "forever" in order to provide her with the benefits of breastmilk if that's all I was able to do. When magically, late one night at the two week mark while warming a bottle, I tried again and she latched on and nursed as if it were all she had ever known. In fact, after that night, she would never take another bottle or pacifier.

I encourage all of the first time moms to believe in yourselves and your God-given abilities to give birth. Trust your gut and your instincts and surround yourselves with positive, encouraging people. Never underestimate the power of support. It made all the difference in the world for me and made Caroline's birth an experience I'll treasure forever.

Cary & Steve Odom

It's So Easy

"It's so easy when you have an epidural." This was what most of my neighbors said about their childbirth experiences. One neighbor reacted differently, however, and suggested we attend prepared childbirth classes. Our first Lamaze experience was great. We liked the classes and the new friends, especially since we all shared an impending joy. I guess we were not really dedicated to "going natural" since we knew that the epidural was so easy if I needed it. Also it was hard to imagine that these breathing techniques could really help you. And how bad could the contractions be? But once again, if I couldn't handle it, it was no problem, the epidural was so easy. Wrong! I went into labor a month early with no time to practice. My labor seemed to progress well and I was "handling" the contractions. When things did get rough, however, I had the epidural. We didn't know until later that we were well in transition and close to pushing. The epidural lowered my blood pressure, stopped my contractions, and probably prolonged my labor by several hours.

When our lovely daughter was two years old, we ventured into Lamaze classes again. This time we had a quiet determination to have an unmedicated delivery and to be more prepared. We listened a little closer. We asked more questions. We studied the breathing techniques more and were really excited about the variations. It gave us some alternatives that we could adjust to our needs. We were ready when our son came two weeks early. This time we knew exactly what stage of labor we were in and used all prepared techniques as planned. Our son was born "naturally." Everything was so much better with prepared childbirth. The delivery was easier and the recovery was much quicker. We were so prepared that we were even going to video tape the birth. Our hospital had just allowed video cameras in the delivery room. I was ready to push when we discovered that we had left the camera in the labor room. My doctor, anxious to be a part of this new experience, sent someone for the camera and told me to keep blowing! I kept blowing. It was no problem. After all, "It's so easy" when you're prepared!

Buffie, Tom, Dawn, & Dane Davenport

The Long and Short Of It

After giving birth for the second time, I was amazed at how different two labors could be. I wouldn't trade the experience of either of them, because each brought us a baby – the most precious gift in the world.

With our first child our story began on a Tuesday, four days before our due date. I was upset when my doctor informed me that day that it would be one to two weeks before I would deliver. I decided to try to change that prediction, so for the next two nights Larry and I played tennis. Perhaps that did the trick, for at 6 a.m. on Thursday I lost my mucus plug and my contractions began.

At noon my contractions were ten minutes apart and easy to handle. By 6 p.m. they still did not require much concentration, but I was certainly aware they were there – every five to seven minutes. Larry and I decided to have supper just in case we were going to need the energy later. Although these contractions had been going on all day, I kept telling myself this was false labor—but it wasn't. From 9 p.m. to midnight, contractions came every three minutes and lasted ninety seconds. This had to be labor. We called the doctor and went to the hospital. The nurse checked me and I was only 2 centimeters dilated and 90% effaced. Oh, how disappointing! Contractions all day and only 2 cm. We decided to walk and walk and walk. A check at 4 a.m. told us the baby was posterior and I was only 3-4 cm. dilated. I was having back labor. There was pain in my back even when there were no contractions. Time was passing slowly, contractions were getting harder, and I was losing my concentration. I was given some medication to help me relax. Larry applied counterpressure to my low back and gave me lots of encouragement, though he too was exhausted. I told him I could not take any more, but he told me I could—and I did. At 7 a.m. the baby still had not turned, but I had made it to 9 cm. At full dilation, I had no urge to push, making it difficult to do so. With the support of my husband and doctor I did get the baby pushed down enough for her to be manually rotated. It then took about ten more hard pushing contractions before our 8 pound-14½ ounce daughter, Holly

Rene, was born. It was a long and difficult labor, but Holly was worth it.

As Larry and I were adjusting to being parents, we found out it wouldn't be long until we were parents of two. Believe me, nursing your baby does not prevent you from getting pregnant. I was due again fourteen months after Holly's birth.

The day before this due date the doctor told me I was 2 cm. dilated and 60% effaced. He said I would probably go another week before delivery. This time I did not play tennis, but that night I did not sleep well due to some strong Braxton-Hicks contractions. By 10 a.m., I was deciding perhaps these were true contractions, so I finished the laundry, packed, and left for the doctor's office. My doctor said I was 3 cm. dilated, and 80% effaced. He gave us the choice of going home to wait or going to the hospital for him to break my bag of waters to see if labor would pick up. We opted for the latter. When my water was broken there was no immediate change in my contractions. I was 4 cm. and a minus 3 station. An hour later I was 6 cm. and a minus 1 station. Things certainly were progressing faster than last time! I began to need the breathing techniques around 3:30 when I was about 7 cm. dilated. How different than before. I had decided that this time I was going to sit up or walk as long as I possibly could in hopes this would give me that *urge* to push. During transition I was able to relax and knew all that was going on around me. This baby, too, was posterior – I guess that's the way I carry babies. My doctor had me lie on my side to help the baby turn. I then needed Larry to give some counter pressure during some of the contractions, though it was nothing like the back labor I'd had before. At 4:30, I was 8 cm. and had a small urge to push. Five minutes later I was 10 cm. and *the urge* arrived in full force. The birthing bed was made ready for delivery. It was good to be in control with gentle pushing. No episiotomy was necessary. The sensation of giving birth was marvelous once again.

Shelly & Larry Eswein

A Special Delivery

One morning in the middle of April, I awoke and blurted out to my husband that the previous night I had gotten pregnant. He looked at me, laughed…mumbled something about a vivid imagination and totally dis-

missed the subject. Four weeks later, after a visit to my OB-GYN, I walked into his office and announced that the rabbit had died. From then on, (at least where my pregnancy was concerned) I was convinced I was psychic. It was just a matter of patience now, after all "Madame Lorie" knew that in nine months she would be giving birth to a beautiful baby boy and have the smoothest delivery ever to be recorded in medical archives.

My pregnancy was literally textbook. A little morning sickness in the second and third month, but aside from that, I was your typical radiant and happy pregnant lady. I quit my job in my fourth month…basked in my husband's attention and read everything even remotely connected with my condition and babies. From the beginning I wanted to attempt an unmedicated birth and was determined to be as well prepared as possible. In my seventh month, Chris (my husband) and I registered for our Lamaze classes where we learned to pelvic-tilt, breathe, and Kegel the rest of my pregnancy away.

On my due date, January 8th, I was informed by my doctor that most likely I'd be about a week late. The baby was in position but had not dropped yet and by my calculations that seemed about right. So that day I went home planning to go shopping the next day for slippers to match the robe I had gotten for Christmas.

Saturday, January 9th, I awoke at 5:00 a.m. with a very strong cramping sensation in my lower abdomen. I went to the bathroom thinking it would probably stop momentarily…it did…five minutes later it returned. By 5:30, I woke Chris up and made the intelligent statement that I didn't know what was happening but whatever it was, it was happening every 5 minutes. We called the doctor who advised us to go to the hospital.

"No, no!" I kept thinking, this isn't the way it's going to be. Where was my quiet time? I was supposed to be playing cards…watching TV…relaxing…and anyway I wasn't going to have my baby for another week. I refused to call the sensations I was experiencing "labor," and was sure they'd send me back from the hospital despite the strength of my contractions. Vanity above everything, I insisted on showering and washing my hair before leaving and, oh yes, packing my suitcase.

At 8:00 a.m. we arrived at the hospital, and by 8:05 were officially told that I was in labor. At my arrival I was 3 cm. dilated and when my doctor came in an hour later I was up to 4 cm.

Once in the hospital and convinced I was actually in labor, we really started to work. Side by side we walked up and down the corridor. The contractions were coming strong and steady – about every 3 minutes – and I really had to breathe to get through them; but we were handling it well. We couldn't help but be somewhat disappointed when at noon the doctor announced I was still at 4 cm.

Around 1:30 p.m., he decided to break my water. On doing this, he observed signs of meconium, so I was connected to a fetal monitor, where the electrode is applied to the baby's scalp. Being on the monitor was uncomfortable mostly because it limited me to, at best, a semi-reclining position, but it was worth it to know that my baby was in no immediate danger. An hour later, still at 4 cm. the doctor suggested pitocin, hoping that it would get me to dilate. The pitocin was administered through an IV that was hooked up earlier. My contractions had been strong since the beginning of my labor, growing with intensity and duration by the hour. After the pitocin, however, I felt close to despair. I couldn't concentrate on my focal point and the contractions seemed to be taking over my entire body. My husband came to the rescue. He gently but firmly talked me into relaxing and breathed with me until slowly I began regaining control. At 4:30 p.m., still at 4 cm., my doctor came in and said the word I thought I'd never heaR – Cesarean. Chris and I had been looking forward to a totally natural birthing experience…but by this point our main concern was having a healthy baby. For some reason I was not dilating, despite having been in active labor for 10 hours, and because of the meconium, there was an added risk. All I wanted was for something to happen. By 5:00 p.m. I had been prepped, given an epidural, and wheeled into the operating room. Chris left my side only long enough to suit up. When he walked in and sat by me I looked into his eyes and smiled. A feeling of peace and confidence that we had made the right decision overcame me and from that moment on I knew everything would be fine.

Soon our little person came into the world protesting loudly the release from the womb that had reluctantly let go. Almost miraculously, the minute Chris cradled and talked to our child, the cries ceased. I felt drunk and giddy with joy…we were finally three. So at 5:46 p.m. another one of my famous predictions came true…. I had a beautiful baby, the only slight deviation was that we had to call her Jessica instead of James.

Just a few end notes. I breastfed my baby in the recovery room and we established a beautiful nursing relationship from day one. Jessica is a happy and healthy child bringing into our lives more happiness than we thought possible. My recovery from surgery was very fast and in six weeks (thanks to nursing) I had lost 30 of the 40 lbs. I gained during pregnancy. I lost those last 10 lbs. too, but I still don't have a pair of slippers to match the robe I got for Christmas.

Lorie & Chris Roberts

A Proud Grandma's Story

I want to share with you a love story!

Five days ago, I became the grandmother of the most precious little boy on earth! Juan Manuel, arrived two weeks early taking us all by surprise.

His birth has been the most amazing and memorable experience that I have witnessed in recent times. It can only be compared to what I felt at the births of my daughters. It has touched and changed my life forever.

It was truly a labor of love, into which my daughter surrendered, listening to her body, and trusting it completely. Even when some of those around her doubted that a natural birth would be possible, she acted with great confidence and ability, showing them otherwise. She never lost her good nature and sense of humor. After 40 hours of very hard work (two days and two nights) she triumphantly came out of this experience feeling on top of the world, more mature and womanly than I could have ever imagined. Here was this girl who dreaded shots, cried like a baby at the sight of a syringe, and made such a huge fuss about them, working beautifully through huge contractions with a persistent posterior presentation that never rotated no matter what she tried and, as you might have guessed, a bad case of back labor. She never complained about the long hours or the grueling pain. Her only concern was for her baby and her fears of ending with a cesarean or huge interventions.

Fortunately, her obstetrician never gave up on her, and sat by her side waiting for nature to take its course. After being stuck for three hours at 7 cm., she was finally completely dilated within the next hour. Almost three hours of pushing later, little Juan Manuel was born facing his mother (posterior) and with his fist on his chin. He was crying even before leaving his mother's body, but when placed on his mom's belly the cries changed into suckling sounds as he licked his mother's breast and found his way to her nipple.

At that exact moment I thanked God from the bottom of my heart for the incredible miracle that I had just witnessed. There are no words to describe what I felt a few moments later when my son-in-law, tears rolling down his face, placed my grandson in my arms and he gazed straight into my eyes.

It has been a unique and wonderful privilege to have served my daughter as her doula. I feel honored and blessed for this opportunity. I have witnessed an incredible transformation in my daughter as she entered motherhood. My admiration, respect and love for her grow indefinitely. I am sure they will be the best parents and the most loving!

Elena Carrillo
The proudest grandma in the world

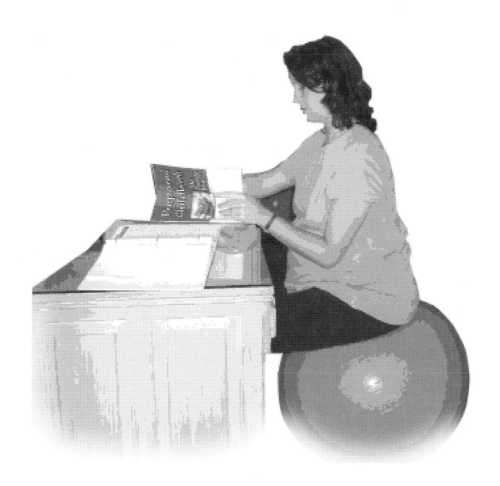

Workbook

For Practice and Review

Practice Page

To derive the greatest benefit from both this book and your childbirth classes, you should spend some time each week in practice. The birth fitness exercises will help you feel better by relieving backache, aiding circulation, and increasing flexibility. Relaxation techniques should be practiced after they have been demonstrated to you in class. They may be learned in any order. These stress reduction skills may be used in many life situations. Breathing patterns are taught to enhance relaxation and concentration. Using different positions for comfort, practice various breathing patterns each week as they are demonstrated so you will feel comfortable using them. Partners who practice together will find it easier to identify and release tension and to concentrate on the familiar breathing patterns when labor occurs. You will feel like a team prepared for birth.

Use the following chart to make sure you do the assignments and practice all the skills covered in class each week. Blanks have been left in case your childbirth educator has additional skills she would like for you to practice.

		Week 1	Week 2	Week 3	Week 4	Week 5 & After
General	Mom and partner read ***Prepared Childbirth – The Family Way***					
	Use good *Body Mechanics* – pg. 12-13					
	Wellness Goals for Pregnancy – pg. 84					
	Nutrition Crossword Puzzle – pg. 89					
	Complete the *Diet Evaluation* – pg. 91					
	How Well Do You Know Your Body? – pg. 87					
	Pain Medication Preference Scale – pg. 98					
	Pack your goody bag – pg. 84					
Exercises	*Birth Fitness Exercises* – pgs. 14-15 & 18-19					
	Kegel Exercises – pg. 16					
	Fun and Fast Format for Feeling Fit and Flexible – pg. 88					
	Walking or other aerobic exercise – pg. 17					
Relaxation & Breathing	Review *Active Relaxation Techniques* (overview) – pgs. 22-24					
	Progressive Tense/Release Practice – pg. 92					
	Touch Relaxation – pg. 24					
	Relaxing Words – pg. 93					
	Relaxing Images – pg. 94					
	Slow Paced Breathing – pg. 39					
	Modified Paced Breathing – pg. 39					
	Practice Rhythmic Breathing – pg. 95					
	With This Birth, I Plan to Try – pg. 96					

What to Pack

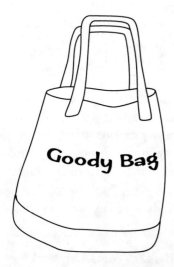

Goody Bag
For Labor

_____ This handbook

_____ Robe and slippers for walking during labor

_____ Focal point(s)

_____ Favorite music with portable CD or tape player

_____ Sour candy on a stick

_____ Flavorings for ice chips

_____ Colored washcloths

_____ Lotion or oil for massage (scented, if you like)

_____ Chapstick/lipstick

_____ Mouthwash and/or toothbrush and toothpaste

_____ Deck of cards, magazine, book

_____ Nutritious snack for partner

_____ Contact lens case and eyeglasses

_____ Warm socks

_____ One or more items for back massage

_____ Vibrating pillow and/or vibrating massager

_____ List of phone numbers and people to notify of the birth (including your childbirth educator)

_____ Change for phone or vending machine

_____ Band for long hair

_____ Fan

_____ Hand mirror to view pushing in the labor room

_____ Paper and pencil

_____ Camera and/or video recorder

_____ Extra pillows with colored pillowcases

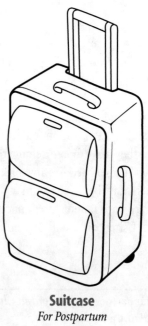

Suitcase
For Postpartum

_____ Two or three nightgowns.

_____ Robe

_____ Slippers

_____ Two or three bras.

If you are planning to nurse:

___ nursing bras (you will probably need a full cup size larger than you wore before becoming pregnant)

___ nursing pads (cloth or paper)

___ a good breastfeeding book

___ nursing gowns (it is nice to have gowns with hidden openings in the front)

_____ Toilet articles

_____ Hair care items

_____ Cosmetics

_____ Going home outfit for mom–early pregnancy size

_____ Going home outfit and blanket for baby

_____ A good book

_____ Baby book (for footprints)

_____ Inexpensive watch or clock

_____ Birth announcements, if desired

_____ Small change

_____ Labor and Birth Questionnaire (page 103)

Also
For the Ride Home

_____ Infant carseat

Wellness Goals for Pregnancy

	Mom's Goals	Target Date	Progress
Nutrition			
Exercise			
Stress Management Techniques			
Other			

	Partner's Goals	Target Date	Progress
Nutrition			
Exercise			
Stress Management Techniques			
Other			

Counting Fetal Movements

Fetal movement is one indication of the baby's well-being. A noticeable decrease or sudden change in fetal movements may indicate that your baby needs additional testing. Some caregivers ask that all pregnant women chart fetal movements after the 32nd week of pregnancy, while others ask only high-risk pregnant women to do so. Many women find that charting fetal movements is enjoyable and allows them special time to focus on their babies and notice their levels of activity. Other women may find charting fetal movements worrisome. Feel free to discuss with your caregiver his or her recommendation for you.

One of the most popular methods of counting fetal movements is the "Count-to-Ten" method. Set aside a time to count fetal movements and begin counting when the baby is awake and active. Consider a kick, wiggle, twist, or a long, continuous roll as one movement. Do not count hiccups as movements. Wait for a pause in activity to count it as one movement. The pause may last as little as a few seconds to more than an hour if the baby falls asleep.

Place an "X" on the chart to note the time the first movement begins. Begin counting and again mark the chart when you feel the tenth fetal movement. In the example, the first fetal movement began at 10:30 a.m. and the tenth fetal movement was felt at 1:00 p.m. Do not be alarmed if the time required to reach ten movements varies from day to day. The time will vary each day due to fetal sleep/awake cycles. Call your caregiver *immediately* if you have not counted ten movements within four hours after the beginning of the first movement or, over a period of several days, you find that it is taking longer and longer to complete ten movements.

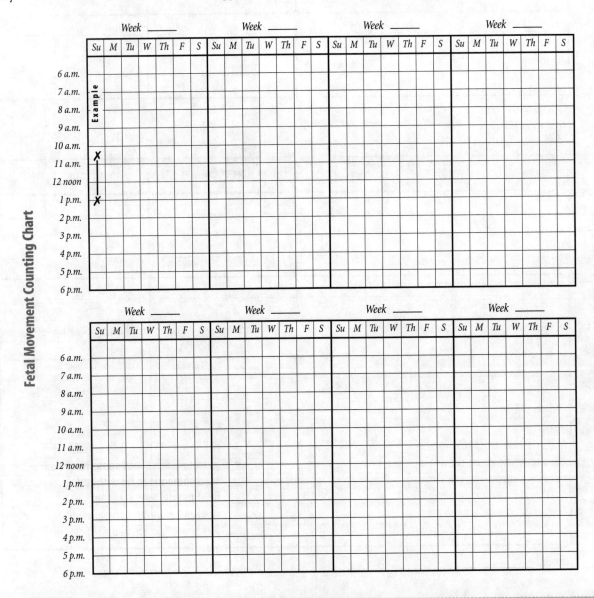

Fetal Movement Counting Chart

How Well Do You Know Your Body?

<table>
<tr><td align="center">**Mom**</td><td align="center">**Partner**</td></tr>
</table>

When I am tense or under stress, I feel tension in my	**When I am tense or under stress, I feel tension in my**
_____ head	_____ head
_____ jaws	_____ jaws
_____ neck	_____ neck
_____ shoulders	_____ shoulders
_____ chest	_____ chest
_____ stomach	_____ stomach
_____ back	_____ back
_____ other _____	_____ other _____
My body reacts to tension by	**My body reacts to tension by**
_____ sweating	_____ sweating
_____ heart rate increasing	_____ heart rate increasing
_____ heart pounding	_____ heart pounding
_____ difficulty catching breath	_____ difficulty catching breath
_____ clammy skin	_____ clammy skin
_____ trembling hands or legs	_____ trembling hands or legs
_____ "butterflies" in stomach	_____ "butterflies" in stomach
_____ nausea	_____ nausea
_____ gripping fists	_____ gripping fists
_____ itching/scratching	_____ itching/scratching
_____ pumping top leg when legs crossed	_____ pumping top leg when legs crossed
_____ biting nails	_____ biting nails
_____ grinding teeth	_____ grinding teeth
_____ speech difficulties	_____ speech difficulties
_____ other _____	_____ other _____
I can recognize signs of tension in my body by	**I can recognize signs of tension in my body by**
_____	_____
_____	_____
I can prevent tension from overwhelming me by	**I can prevent tension from overwhelming me by**
_____	_____
_____	_____
I use the following calming techniques when needed	**I use the following calming techniques when needed**
_____ paced breathing	_____ paced breathing
_____ consciously relaxing all muscle groups	_____ consciously relaxing all muscle groups
_____ imagery	_____ imagery
_____ other _____	_____ other _____
To cope with pain, I	**To cope with pain, I**
_____ need quiet to tune into myself	_____ need quiet to tune into myself
_____ need to think about something else	_____ need to think about something else
_____ need someone to be with me	_____ need someone to be with me
_____ need to talk with someone	_____ need to talk with someone
_____ need to be doing something	_____ need to be doing something
_____ want help from a medical person	_____ want help from a medical person
_____ want to be alone	_____ want to be alone
_____ other _____	_____ other _____

Fun and Fast Format for Feeling Fit and Flexible

Head to toe in 5 minutes or more.

Remember to:

- Use slow, controlled movements when stretching; never bounce or jerk.
- Work to feel stretch, not pain.
- Hold a stretch from 20 seconds to a minute or more to benefit from it.
- Exhale as you go into the stretch, then breathe normally.
- Feel the release of tension as you allow the muscle to relax.
- Actively feel the stretch in your muscles, not joints.

Head and Neck

- Look far right; hold; center; far left; hold; center; repeat.
- Drop right ear to right shoulder; hold; drop left ear to left shoulder; hold; drop chin to chest; hold; repeat.

Shoulders, Arms, Hands

- Holding arms out shoulder level make small, then large circles in a spiral. Circle forward then reverse.
- Lift elbows up to shoulder level with fingers and fore-arms pointing down; bending elbows, bring tightened fists in towards face; then straighten elbows, stretching arms and fingers out shoulder level. Repeat in and out picturing your arms as windshield wipers.

Back, Abdominals, Pelvic Floor

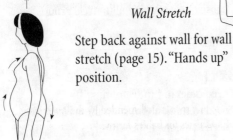

Wall Stretch

Step back against wall for wall stretch (page 15). "Hands up" position.

Standing Pelvic Tilt

Standing pelvic tilt (page 14). Add Kegel while in tilt (page 16).

Wall Squat

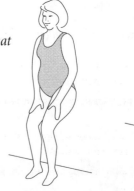
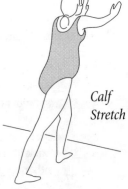

Calf Stretch

Legs

- *Wall Squat* – squat down; hold to feel tension in thighs; breathe through "pain" (page 15).
- *Calf Stretch* – turn to face wall; stretch (page 15).
- *Ankle Rotation* – Hold on to wall or partner if needed for support and lift foot for ankle rotation.

Feet

- Standing foot stretch (do not curl toes). Pull ball of foot toward heel, raising arch. Release, repeat.

Body Stretch with Posture Check

- Stand tall dropping shoulders with arms at your side, then raise both arms straight overhead and stretch; lower arms to shoulder level, palms facing up; then, press arms back 5 times, pinching shoulder blades together with each press. Replace arms to your sides.
- Rub hands together to warm; place hands over eyes; rock gently forward and back on your feet until you "settle." Remove hands from eyes; drop shoulders, hands at side. Feel your body's posture. Relax head, eyes, jaws, shoulders, chest (big relaxing breath), re-lease abdominal muscles, hips; feel tension flow all the way out your toes.
- Open eyes; feel refreshed, flexible and "in line."

This sequence may be done all at one time, or the various exercises may be spaced out through a day as you feel the need to stretch or unwind. Adapt these and other movements on pages 14-17 to sitting at a desk, in a car or plane, or even in bed before getting up. Add a walk around the block, a bike ride, swim or other aerobic exercise to your daily routine. You will feel better when you feel fit and flexible!

Nutrition Crossword Puzzle

Across

1. You can easily combine grains and vegetables into a hearty
   _____.

3. Because vitamins B and C are not stored by the body, how often
   do you need to consume them?

5. Especially in pregnancy, it is dangerous to eat meat that is too
   _____.

6. A nickname for the classification of foods that supplies the most
   easily used form of energy for the body.

7. The "almost perfect" food that supplies protein, calcium, phos-
   phorus, and vitamin D.

8. In addition to water, a recommended beverage.

9. Most nutritionists believe that small amounts of Nutrasweet are
   _____ during pregnancy.

10. The minimum number of recommended daily servings from
    the grains food group.

11. Nutrition for the pregnant woman is especially important in the
    last three months of pregnancy because critical development is
    taking place in the baby's _____.

12. A carbohydrate or protein provides four calories per gram while
    a _____ provides nine calories per gram.

14. The factor which many believe may contribute most to the
    development of a healthy baby.

16. For heart-healthy eating, choose this kind of milk.

17. A beverage *not* recommended during pregnancy.

21. A seasoning many *wrongly* believe should be restricted during
    pregnancy.

22. For heart-healthy eating, choose this kind of meat, poultry, or
    fish.

23. Adding nuts, raisins, and whole grains to _____ dough can
    make these a healthy snack.

25. At least _____ glasses of water are recommended daily during
    pregnancy.

28. Beans, nuts, whole grains and dairy products can be combined
    to provide protein sources which could substitute for _____.

29. Weight gain of approximately _____ pound(s) per week
    during the last three months of pregnancy is(are) recommend-
    ed.

30. When eating "fast-foods," include a _____ with your meal to
    add valuable nutrients.

Down

2. A pregnant woman needs 60 grams of _____ each day.

3. Thiamin, a B vitamin, is called the "morale vitamin" because a
   deficiency may cause _____.

4. Liver; dairy products; dark-green, orange and deep _____
   vegetables are excellent sources of vitamin A.

13. No more than _____ percent of your daily calories should
    come from fats.

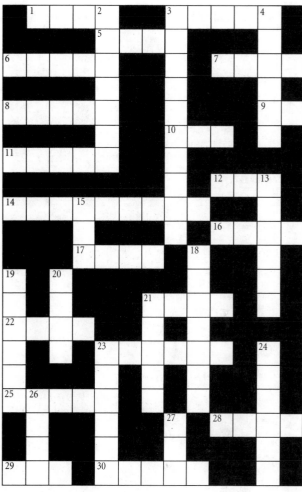

15. Fruits and vegetables provide the most nutrients when eaten
    _____ or steamed.

18. A meal with broccoli, cheese sauce, canned salmon, and milk
    is very high in this mineral.

19. Green leafy and dark yellow fruits and vegetables are excellent
    sources of this important B vitamin, an essential component
    of blood cells.

20. This nutrient can be added to foods or eaten alone to add fiber
    to the diet.

21. Babies who are exposed to _____ are more likely to develop
    respiratory problems during the first year of life.

23. Green peppers, tomatoes, broccoli, strawberries, and _____
    fruits are good sources of vitamin C.

24. The type of feeding most recommended by the American
    Academy of Pediatrics for babies for the first year of life.

26. The body's demand for this mineral during pregnancy is so
    high that it is difficult to meet the daily requirement by diet
    alone.

27. Drinking _____ inhibits the absorption of iron from food
    eaten at the same meal.

Protein, Calorie, and Fat Counter

Dairy Products:	Protein(g)	Calories	%Fat
Butter, 1 tbsp.	Trace	102	100
Margarine, 1 tbsp.	Trace	101	100
†Milk:			
Whole, 1 cup	8	150	49
Skim, 1 cup	8	86	4.2
†Cheese:			
Cheddar, 1 oz.	7	114	74
American, 1 oz.	6	105	75
Cottage, creamed, ½ cup	13	108	39
Cream, 1 oz.	2	98	88
Swiss, 1 oz.	8	105	66
†Yogurt, fruit, lowfat, 1 cup	9	240	11
Vanilla Ice Cream, ½ cup	2	140	45
Vanilla Shake (Burger King)	9	321	28
✓†Eggs, one	6	79	64
Meat, Poultry, Fish:			
Beef:			
Chuck, pot roast, 3 oz.	22	278	66
Hamburger, 70% lean, 3 oz.	21	246	64
Hamburger, 80% lean, 3 oz.	21	231	61
Roast, lean, 3 oz.	23	209	53
Steak, sirloin, lean, 3 oz.	26	180	40
Steak, round, lean, 3 oz.	24	165	38
Corned, 3 oz.	15	213	68
Chipped, creamed, 5 oz.	11	160	51
Stew, with vegetables, 1 cup	16	218	45
Bologna, 2 slices	5	144	84
Chicken:			
Breast, roasted, 3½ oz.	29	193	35
Breast, fried, 3½ oz.	31	218	36
Duck, 3 oz.	16	286	76
Lamb:			
Chop, broiled, 3 oz.	24	159	36
Leg, roasted, 3 oz.	26	177	39
✓Liver:			
Beef, 3 oz.	21	137	28
Chicken, 3 oz.	21	133	32
Liverwurst, 1 slice	3	59	78
Pork:			
Bacon, crisp, 2 slices	4	72	78
Chop, 3 oz.	25	301	64
Ham steak, lean, 3 oz.	17	105	31
Ham, luncheon meat, 1 slice	5	52	52
Hot dog, one	5	144	81
Sausage, 1 piece	12	200	72
Turkey, light, 3 oz.	24	167	38
Veal:			
Cutlet, broiled, 3 oz.	23	185	46
Fish:			
Haddock, fried, 3 oz.	16	194	45
Fish sticks, breaded, 2 medium	9	155	41
Shrimp, broiled, 3 oz.	18	84	10
Tuna, packed in water, 3 oz.	23	110	16
✓Nuts and Seeds:			
†Almonds, 1 oz.	4	165	81
Peanuts, 1 oz.	8	162	77
Peanut butter, 2 tbsp.	9	190	76
Pecans, 1 oz.	2	185	88
Sunflower seeds, 1 oz.	5	163	77
Dried Beans:			
Lima, cooked, ½ cup	7	108	3
Navy, cooked, ½ cup	8	112	4
Kidney, canned, ½ cup	7	102	4
Grains (whole grains):			
Biscuits, one	2	103	42
Bread: white or wholewheat, 1 slice	2	65	14
Cereal, oatmeal, 1 oz.	5	110	16
Cereal, Rice Krispies, 1 oz.	2	110	0
Pasta (rotini), 2 oz.	7	210	4
Rice, white, 1½ cup	3	131	2
Rolls, dinner, one	2	85	21
Cornbread, one	4	198	33
Saltines, five	1	52	24

Vegetables:	Protein(g)	Calories	%Fat
✓Asparagus, cooked, ½ cup	2	22	0
Beans:			
Green, cooked, ½ cup	1	22	0
✓Lima, cooked, ½ cup	7	94	0
✓†Broccoli*, cooked, ½ cup	2	23	0
✓Brussels sprouts, cooked, ½ cup	2	30	0
†Cabbage*:			
Coleslaw, 1 serving	2	119	50
Cooked, ½ cup	1	16	0
Carrots, raw, ½ cup	1	31	0
Corn, cooked, ½ cup	3	89	10
Lettuce, leaf, ½ cup	1	5	0
Peas, cooked, ½ cup	3	67	0
Pepper, bell*, chopped, ½ cup	Trace	19	0
✓Potatoes:			
Baked (with skin on*) 1 medium	5	218	0
French fries, 10	2	158	47
Mashed, ½ cup	2	111	36
Chips, 1 oz.	2	150	60
✓†Spinach, cooked, ½ cup	3	21	0
Tomato*, raw, 1 medium	1	24	0
Fruits:			
Apple, 1 medium	Trace	81	0
✓Avocado, ½ large	2	153	88
Banana, 1 medium	1	109	0
✓Cantaloupe*, ½ medium	2	90	0
Grapefruit*, ½	1	38	0
Grapes, Concord ½ cup	Trace	29	0
Orange*, 1 medium	1	62	0
✓†Orange juice*, 1 cup (calcium fortified)	2	112	6.4
Peach, fresh, 1 medium	1	37	0
Pear, fresh, 1 medium	1	97	0
Pineapple, fresh, ½ cup	Trace	38	0
Plum, 1 medium	1	36	0
Prune juice, 1 cup	2	182	1.6
Raisins, ½ cup	0	217	0
✓Strawberries*, raw, 1 cup	1	45	0
✓Watermelon, diced, ½ cup	1	26	0
Beverages (other):			
Coffee, black, 6 oz.	0	11	0.8
Beer, 12 oz.	1	146	0
Wine, red, 3½ oz.	Trace	74	0
Whiskey, gin, rum, vodka, 1 oz.	0	105	0
Desserts and Sweets:			
Cake:			
Chocolate with icing, 1 slice	2	169	39
Angel food, 1 slice	4	143	1
Doughnut, plain, one	3	210	51
Pie:			
Apple, 1 slice	3	302	39
Custard, 1 slice	6	207	46
Fast Foods:			
McDonald's Big Mac	25	560	52
Burger King hamburger	15	344	29
McDonald's Filet-O-Fish	14	440	53
Long John Silver's fish, 1 piece, 3 oz.	13	202	53
Kentucky Fried Chicken, breast	26	257	49
Pizza Hut cheese pizza –			
½ of 10" pie (thin crust)	25	450	30
Taco Bell taco	10	184	54
Dairy Queen hot dog	11	280	49
Burger King french fries	4	341	53
McDonald's Egg McMuffin	18	290	35
Other:			
Instant Breakfast, 1 dry, chocolate	4	130	7
Soup:			
Split pea, 1 cup	9	164	16
Cream of broccoli, 1 cup	7	140	39
Vegetable, 1 cup	4	122	27
Chicken noodle, 1 cup	4	72	30

*Good sources of vitamin C †Foods high in calcium ✓Foods high in folic acid

Diet Evaluation

To determine if your diet contains adequate servings of foods from the *Food Guide Pyramid* (page 9), use this form to analyze your diet for any 24 hour period. Your partner might also want to analyze his diet, as the two of you will be setting the nutritional standards in your home for years to come. List all foods, including snacks.

Mother-To-Be/Nursing Mother

Breakfast	Lunch	Dinner	Snacks	Totals
				Basic food group servings:
				Breads, etc. (6 to 11) _____
				Vegetables (3 to 5) _____
				Fruits (2 to 4) _____
				Dairy (3) _____
				Meats, etc. (3) _____
				Fats & sweets (sparingly) _____
				Water (8 + glasses) _____
				Grams of protein: _____
				Calories: _____

Partner

Breakfast	Lunch	Dinner	Snacks	Totals
				Basic food group servings:
				Breads, etc. (6 to 11) _____
				Vegetables (3 to 5) _____
				Fruits (2 to 4) _____
				Dairy (2-3) _____
				Meats, etc. (2-3) _____
				Fats & sweets (sparingly) _____
				Water (8 + glasses) _____
				Grams of protein: _____
				Calories: _____

General Guidelines – The recommended daily allowance (RDA) for calories for pregnant women is 2500, for breastfeeding mothers is 2700, for active men is 2800, and for nonpregnant active women is 2200. The RDA for grams of protein is 60 for pregnant women, 65 for breastfeeding mothers (first 6 months), 62 for breastfeeding mothers (second 6 months), 58 to 63 for men, and 46 to 50 for nonpregnant women. The 1990 Dietary Guidelines recommend that all Americans (over the age of two) limit fat in their diets to 30% of daily calories.

Progressive Tense/Release Practice

By practicing the following tension awareness exercise, you will learn to recognize tension as it builds in your body throughout the day. By listening to your body you may be able to release that tension before it turns to pain.

For each part of your body:

- First, think about how the muscle group feels now.
- Then, tighten – contract or stretch the muscle group; and
- Hold to a count of 5 as you concentrate on what you feel; study the sensation when the muscle is tight.
- Finally, release the tension to a count of 10, let go; compare the difference between feelings of tension and release.

Muscle	Tighten or Stretch	Hold & Concentrate	Release/Relax
Forehead	Raise eyebrows Frown	Hold to a count of 5 & concentrate Hold to a count of 5 & concentrate	Let go, release Smooth the forehead
Eyes	Look up, down, right, left	Hold to a count of 5 & concentrate	Close eyes softly
Mouth	Press lips together Smile (exaggerate) Press tongue against teeth	Hold to a count of 5 & concentrate Hold to a count of 5 & concentrate Hold to a count of 5 & concentrate	Part lips slightly Soften smile Let tongue feel thick
Jaws	Bite teeth together gently Drag jaw down, wide open	Hold to a count of 5 & concentrate Hold to a count of 5 & concentrate	Let jaw fall open slightly Close jaw softly
Neck	Pull head into shoulders like a turtle	Hold to a count of 5 & concentrate	Rotate head on neck
Shoulders	Round shoulders forward Pull shoulders back Pull shoulders down toward feet	Hold to a count of 5 & concentrate Hold to a count of 5 & concentrate Hold to a count of 5 & concentrate	Release to neutral Release to neutral Release to neutral
Arms	Pull tight against body	Hold to a count of 5 & concentrate	Allow to dangle
Hands	Clench fists Stretch fingers long	Hold to a count of 5 & concentrate Hold to a count of 5 & concentrate	Allow fingers to curl gently Release the stretch
Chest	Fill lungs with air	Hold to a count of 5 & concentrate	Let the air out
Abdomen	Pull belly in to hug baby	Hold to a count of 5 & concentrate	Let go of hug
Hips	Pinch buttocks together	Hold to a count of 5 & concentrate	Let muscles spread
Thighs	Push feet and legs together Press hips and knees outward	Hold to a count of 5 & concentrate Hold to a count of 5 & concentrate	Let them flop open Let them go loose
Legs	Flex foot and stretch leg	Hold to a count of 5 & concentrate	Drop foot and leg
Feet	Curl toes gently (do not point)	Hold to a count of 5 & concentrate	Release the curl

Sequence for Learning Progressive Relaxation

1. Progressive tense/release as outlined above.
2. Just think of each muscle listed above, then release that muscle without first tightening or stretching.
3. Think and release in larger groups all at one time:

    head, neck, shoulders, arms...release

    chest, abdomen, back...release

    hips, legs, feet...release

4. Final mastery is when you simply say to yourself, "let go" or "release" and your entire body relaxes!

Relaxing Words

Phrases to Relax With

This is a modified autogenic exercise

I feel very calm and quiet. I close my eyes and focus my awareness inside myself. I deepen my breathing and quiet my thoughts. I let my body be still and my muscles release.

My scalp is loose and relaxed. My head feels comfortable and quiet. My eyes feel heavy. My mouth smiles gently as my lips release. My tongue feels thick and moist. My cheeks are loose and my jaw droops. My face and my forehead are smooth, quiet, comfortable, and very relaxed. My neck is comfortable and still. My shoulders hang loose. My arms are floating and tingling. My fingers are curled and warm. My lungs breathe deeply, slowly, as my chest rises and falls with no effort, no thinking. My body just breathes for me; my heartbeat is strong and regular. My belly is soft, round, and filled with quiet energy. My baby inside is floating and peaceful, strong and healthy, warm, safe, and secure. My hips are loose. My legs are loose, motionless. I feel warmth flowing down into my feet. My legs, knees, and ankles are heavy and loose. Within the center of myself I feel quiet, calm, and peaceful. My baby feels my calmness and shares it.

Words That Are Relaxing to Me

Circle the words you like

loose	free
limp	drained
warm	weak
cool	lax
heavy	rested
light	flabby
floating	slack
tingling	comfy
sagging	cozy
thick	secure
curled	snug
soft	mellow
whole	droopy
peaceful	quiet
calm	flexible
flaccid	_____
relaxed	_____
released	_____

Positive Affirmations

Every day my baby grows stronger and stronger.

I feel calm and at peace with the world.

I breathe energy into my baby.

My baby gives me strength to labor.

My world is safe and secure.

My body is made to give birth.

I am strong and able to birth my baby.

_____

_____

_____

_____

_____

_____

Fill in Relaxing Words You Like to Describe

head	_____
eyes	_____
tongue	_____
mouth	_____
jaw	_____
shoulders	_____
arms	_____
hands	_____
fingers	_____
chest	_____
belly	_____
baby	_____
hips	_____
legs	_____
feet	_____

Relaxing Images

Choose Your Own Journey

When you choose your own journey you are totally in control of your images and thoughts. Fill in the following blanks to record scenes, sensations, and suggestions that are pleasant and relaxing for you. Your journey may be to any real or imaginary place. Pretend that you take with you a magic bag that holds anything you need for your comfort. Where will you go on this journey? _____ When you arrive what do you see? _____ The air around you feels _____ . You are dressed very comfortably in _____ . Notice the colors around you. What colors do you see? _____ Breathe in deeply and smell the fragrance of _____ in the air around you. Enjoy that scent that calms you and makes you feel safe, comfortable. As you walk around, what do you feel beneath your feet? _____ Is it soft, hard, crunchy, warm, cool? _____ What do you see in the distance? _____ What do you see nearby? _____ Is there something near you that you would like to touch, to feel, to experience? _____ What is it like? _____ If you would like, you may touch it. Feel the texture, _____ the temperature, _____ the size _____ and shape _____ . What is the color? _____ Is there any water in your image? If so, use it to help you relax as you see fit. Is it just peaceful to look at or listen to, or do you wish to be in it, or touch it, or to drink from it? Water cools and refreshes. Enjoy water by taste or by sight if it fits into your image. Food and drink are comforting. If you feel like it, you can reach into your magic bag and bring out whatever you would like to eat or drink. You may set a feast in your image or simply sip or snack. What would you have? _____ If you choose to eat or drink, what will it be? _____ Focus on the taste: sweet or savory, _____ the texture: juicy or crisp, _____ the temperature: hot or cold _____ . Enjoy!

Now find a spot in your image to recline. Any props you may need are in your magic bag. Snuggle down, curl up, or stretch out as is most relaxing to you. Feel the sensation of total peace come over your entire body. Listen to the sounds around you. Look at the peaceful scene. Enjoy the colors, the textures you see and touch. Breathe in the calm, refreshing air. Tune in to this feeling. Remember it. You can come back to it at any time.

Use the preceding suggestions to help you write your own very special and quieting journey.

My Journey:

_____

_____

_____

_____

_____

_____

_____

_____

_____

_____

_____

_____

_____

_____

_____

_____

_____

After you write your images, find a comfortable place to replay your journey in your mind. Allow the tension to leave your body as your breathing becomes slow and rhythmical and you transport yourself to your special place. The images you have designed will come alive in your mind and your body will relax. As you conclude your image, begin to move your relaxed body slowly. Take your time returning to full activity, but when you do you will have renewed energy, and a sense of well being.

The more you work with your journey, the faster you can achieve your relaxed state even in distracting and less than comfortable situations. Share your images with your partner so he or she can give you these comforting suggestions during your labor.

Practice Rhythmic Breathing
For Both Slow Paced and Modified Paced Breathing

When either a true contraction or a practice contraction begins,
- take a cleansing breath,
- establish a focal point, and
- begin rhythmic breathing.

Breathe in one or more of the following ways through the contraction:
- **in**hale through nose…exhale **out** through mouth
- **in** through nose…**out** through nose
- **in** through mouth…**out** through mouth

Slow Paced Breathing

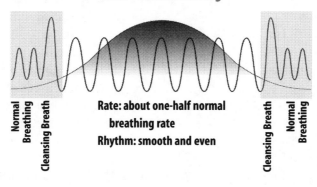

Rate: about one-half normal breathing rate
Rhythm: smooth and even

During a contraction:
- the scene or color I like to visualize is _____
- the phrase I like to say to myself is _____
- the most comfortable number to count to is _____

Modified Paced Breathing

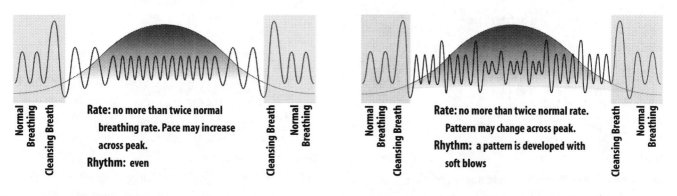

Rate: no more than twice normal breathing rate. Pace may increase across peak.
Rhythm: even

Rate: no more than twice normal rate. Pattern may change across peak.
Rhythm: a pattern is developed with soft blows

During a contraction:
- the scene or color I like to visualize is _____
- the phrase I like to say to myself is _____
- the most comfortable number to count to is _____
- the sound I like to use is _____
- the patterns I like are _____

With This Birth, I Plan to Try

Distractions
_____ Sleep and/or rest
_____ Take a walk
_____ Talk with family and friends
_____ Read
_____ Play a game
_____ Eat a light meal
_____ Breathe in patterns

Relaxation techniques
_____ Use paced breathing
_____ Consciously release each muscle group
_____ Release to partner's touch and/or massage
_____ Use visual imagery

Using the sense of vision
_____ External focal point
_____ Internal focal point

Using the sense of hearing
_____ Play music
_____ Talk
_____ Sing
_____ Read aloud
_____ Moan
_____ Pray
_____ Chant

Using the sense of smell
_____ Pillowcase from home
_____ Washcloth from home
_____ Favorite lotion or fragrance
_____ Baby powder

Using the sense of taste
_____ Popsicles (if available)
_____ Sour sucker
_____ Ice chips with flavorings
_____ Toothpaste and/or mouthwash

Using the sense of touch through temperature
_____ Ice
_____ Heating pad
_____ Hot water bottle
_____ Alternating hot/cold packs
_____ Warmed blankets
_____ Socks
_____ Warm bath and/or shower

Using the sense of touch through movement
_____ Walk
_____ Change positions frequently
_____ Stand
_____ Rock
_____ Hug someone
_____ Slow dance
_____ Do pelvic rock/tilt in all positions
_____ Use patterned breathing
_____ Gently shake joints
_____ Use rhythmical movements
_____ Use the "birth ball" for positioning

Using the sense of touch through steady pressure
_____ Apply chapstick/lipstick
_____ Kiss
_____ Maintain pressure on upper lip with index finger
_____ Use palms to squeeze something
_____ Stand on something hard
_____ Have someone do acupressure
_____ Apply pressure to the external genitalia (sit on an inverted bedpan)

Using the sense of touch on the skin
_____ Lightly stroke sheets with fingertips
_____ Feel partner's face with fingertips
_____ Do light stroking on your belly
_____ Have partner do light stroking on your belly
_____ Partner do gentle touch relaxation

Using the sense of touch through deep pressure and vibration
_____ Sit in a hot tub
_____ Use a shower massage
_____ Use a hot tub foot massager
_____ Use vibrating pillows
_____ Use a vibrating massager
_____ Have someone do acupressure
_____ Partner to massage (heavy pressure)

Other
_____ Partner + additional support person(s)
_____ Doula (professional labor support person)
_____ _____
_____ _____
_____ _____
_____ _____
_____ _____
_____ _____

What Helps Me Relax Best	The Kind of Touch or Massage I Like
Mom	Mom
Partner	Partner

Breathing Strategies I Like	The Kind of Music I Like
Mom	Mom
Partner	Partner

Pain Medications Preference Scale

You and your partner may use this scale to determine your preferences regarding the use of pain medication in labor. Begin with each of you choosing the number that best matches your feelings and then compare. If you are not in close agreement, discuss your reasons and come to an agreement. The pregnant woman's preferences are more important and must prevail if you cannot agree. The right hand column describes what kind of help she needs from her support people.

	What It Means	**How The Partner, Doula, and Caregiver Help**
+10	She wants to feel nothing; desires anesthesia before labor begins.	An impossible extreme. If she has no interest in helping herself in labor, she needs to know she will have pain, and needs reassurance. She should discuss her wishes with her caregiver.
+9	Fear of pain; lack of confidence that she will be able to cope; dependence on staff for pain relief.	Help her accept that she will have some pain. Suggest she discuss fears with caregiver or childbirth educator. She needs information and reassurance, without false expectations.
+7	Definite desire for anesthesia as soon in labor as the doctor will allow it, or before labor becomes painful.	Be sure the caregiver is aware of her desire for early anesthesia and that she knows the potential risks. Learn whether this is possible in your hospital. Inform staff when you arrive.
+5	Desire for epidural anesthesia in active labor (4-5 cm); willingness to cope until then, perhaps with narcotic medication.	Encourage her in breathing and relaxation. Know comfort measures. Suggest medications to her in labor as she approaches active labor.
+3	Desire to use some pain medication, but wants as little as possible; plans to use self-help comfort measures for part of labor.	Plan to help her keep medication use low. Use comfort measures. Help her get medications when she wants them. Suggest reduced doses of narcotics or a "light and late" epidural block.
0	No opinion or preference. This is a rare attitude among pregnant women; but not uncommon among partners or support people.	Become informed. Discuss medications. Help her decide her preferences. If she has no preference ahead of time, follow her wishes during labor.
-3	Prefers that pain medications be avoided, but wants medication as soon as she requests it in labor.	Do not suggest that she take pain medications. Emphasize coping techniques. Do not try to talk her out of pain medications.
-5	Strong preference to avoid pain medications, mainly for benefit to baby and labor progress. Will accept medications for difficult or long labor.	Prepare yourself for a very active role. A doula will be most helpful for both the woman and partner. Know how to help her relax and use the breathing strategies. Know the comfort measures. Do not suggest medications. If she asks, interpret it as a need for more help and try different comfort measures and more intense emotional support first.
-7	Very strong desire for natural childbirth, for sense of personal gratification as well as to benefit baby and labor progress. Will be disappointed if she uses medications.	Follow the recommendations for -5, but with even greater commitment. This means planning not to use pain medications, unless complications develop that require painful procedures, or she is unable to respond to intensive labor support techniques for several contractions in a row. If she asks for medication, plan to encourage alternative comfort measures. You should, however, have a prearranged plan (e.g. a "last resort" code word) for how she can let you know she really has had enough and wants medication.
-9	Wants medication to be denied by staff, even if she asks for it.	This is very difficult for you – to be responsible for her satisfaction. Promise to help all you can, but help her realize the final decision is not yours. It is hers.
-10	Wants no medication, even for cesarean delivery.	An impossible extreme. Encourage her to learn of complications that require painful interventions. Help her get a realistic understanding of risks and benefits of pain medications.

Adapted from: *The Birth Partner: Everything You Need to Know to Help A Woman Through Childbirth,* by Penny Simkin. Harvard Common Press, 1989. Reprinted with permission of the author.

Birth Options

Options to discuss with my partner and healthcare provider:	My ideal labor and birth would include:	If my ideal is not possible, I would like to:	If I need to have a cesarean birth, I would like to:
• Labor support (partner, other family, friend, doula)			
• Spontaneous labor or elective induction			
• Food and fluids by mouth			
• IV or heparin lock			
• Intermittent or continuous monitoring of the fetal heart tones			
• Movement and position changes: walking, slow dancing, rocking chair, birth ball			
• Warm bath/shower during labor			
• Use of comfort techniques: touch and massage, warm and cold packs, aromatherapy			
• Use of analgesia/anesthesia for pain relief			
• Spontaneous or directed pushing, choice of position			
• Perineal massage; routine episiotomy			
• Use of forceps, suction device			
• No separation of mother and baby after birth, or length of time with baby immediately after birth			
• Initiation of breastfeeding			
• Family/sibling visits—rooming in			
• Circumcision; anesthesia for circumcision			

You Know Breastfeeding Is Going Well When . . .

_____ **You recognize your baby's early feeding cues:** Rooting, hand to mouth movements, sucking on hand, small sounds, and small body movements. Crying is a late feeding cue.

_____ **You can nurse comfortably in various positions:** Lying down or sitting with baby in "cradle" or "football" hold.

_____ **Baby is properly positioned when nursing:** Baby's head and shoulders are supported and in a straight line with his body. The baby's head is level with the breast and the baby is turned toward mom so that he can see mom with his top eye.

_____ **You feel comfortable assisting baby to latch-on:** When your nipple lightly touches baby's lips, you wait until the baby opens his mouth wide. You support your breast with one hand (fingers below on ribcage and thumb on top) while using opposite arm to quickly draw baby in when baby's mouth is wide open.

_____ **Baby latches on well:** Takes all of nipple and about one-half to one inch of the areola into his mouth. Lips are flared out and chin and nose are touching the breast.

_____ **You know you are making milk:** In the first week, you may experience uterine cramping each time you nurse; you may get a sleepy feeling; you may notice tingling, pressure, or fullness in the breasts.

_____ **Baby is getting milk:** After a few short fast sucks, you notice a change in pattern to a slow, rhythmic suck-swallow. You can hear the swallow, which sounds like a sigh. When you stop nursing, you can see milk in his mouth and he may spit up some milk when he burps.

_____ **Baby is satisfied:** Your baby is relaxed at the end of the feeding. He may release the breast spontaneously, or he may drift off to sleep after several minutes of active suckling.

_____ **Mother is comfortable after nursing:** After the mature milk comes in, your breasts feel soft and comfortable when your baby finishes nursing. You have no lumps or engorgement.

_____ **Baby nurses at least 8 to 12 times each 24 hours (about every 1½ to 3 hours).**

_____ **Baby has 1 or 2 wet diapers the first day and gradually increases to at least 6 to 8 heavy wet diapers by the end of week one.**

_____ **Baby has 1 or 2 bowel movements the first day and gradually increases to 4 or more per day as the mature milk comes in. The color changes from sticky green-black to a loose, yellow curd-like stool by the end of the first week.**

Note: The amount of urine and stool increases and the frequency decreases as the baby matures. By about 4 weeks, bowel movements may continue as frequently as every feeding or may decrease to large amounts only once a week.

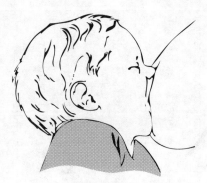

Correct Latch

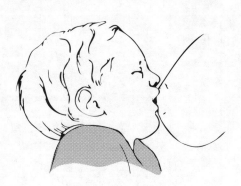

Incorrect Latch

Time Sharing

Mom

This pie represents 24 hours of your day. Draw wedges in the pie to show the number of hours you currently spend in each of your daily activities: eating, cooking, sleeping, at work, grooming, home maintenance/chores, leisure time for self, leisure time for couple, etc.

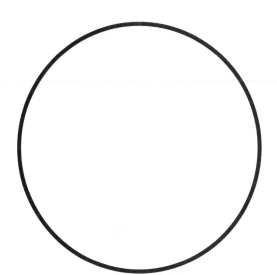

This pie represents 24 hours of your day after your baby arrives. Draw wedges in the pie to show the number of hours you think you will spend in each of your daily activities: eating, sleeping, cooking, at work, grooming, home maintenance/chores, leisure time for self, leisure time for couple, etc. *plus* time spent for baby feeding, laundry, consoling, maintenance, etc.

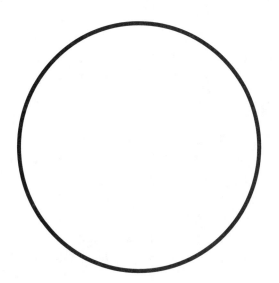

Dad

This pie represents 24 hours of your day. Draw wedges in the pie to show the number of hours you currently spend in each of your daily activities: eating, cooking, sleeping, at work, grooming, home maintenance/chores, leisure time for self, leisure time for couple, etc.

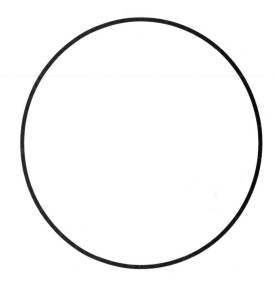

This pie represents 24 hours of your day after your baby arrives. Draw wedges in the pie to show the number of hours you think you will spend in each of your daily activities: eating, sleeping, cooking, at work, grooming, home maintenance/chores, leisure time for self, leisure time for couple, etc. *plus* time spent for baby feeding, laundry, consoling, maintenance, etc.

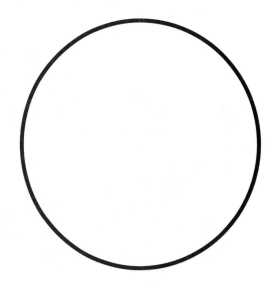

Puzzle Page

Match the following "problems of pregnancy" to the appropriate "comfort measures."
Some may have more than one correct answer.

If you have:

1. leg cramps
2. back-ache
3. incontinence
4. swelling
5. heartburn
6. fatigue
7. constipation
8. hemorrhoids

Then you might try:

a. eat bran/drink water
b. rest/naps
c. calf stretches
d. Kegel exercise
e. sit, swim, or walk in water
f. small, frequent meals
g. posture and position
h. pelvic tilts

UNSCRAMBLE the following words for ideas of things to try in labor, then place the numbered letter in the appropriate boxes for more good advice!

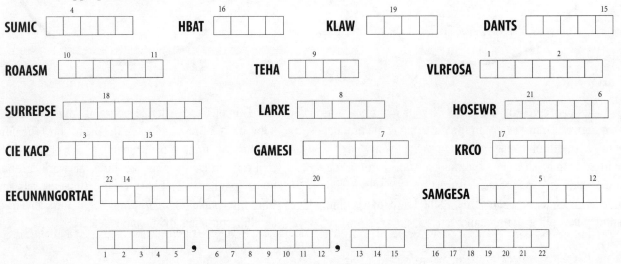

SUMIC ⬜⬜⬜⬜ (4)   HBAT ⬜⬜⬜⬜ (16)   KLAW ⬜⬜⬜⬜ (19)   DANTS ⬜⬜⬜⬜⬜ (15)

ROAASM ⬜⬜⬜⬜⬜⬜ (10, 11)   TEHA ⬜⬜⬜⬜ (9)   VLRFOSA ⬜⬜⬜⬜⬜⬜⬜ (1, 2)

SURREPSE ⬜⬜⬜⬜⬜⬜⬜⬜ (18)   LARXE ⬜⬜⬜⬜⬜ (8)   HOSEWR ⬜⬜⬜⬜⬜⬜ (21, 6)

CIE KACP ⬜⬜⬜ ⬜⬜⬜⬜ (3, 13)   GAMESI ⬜⬜⬜⬜⬜⬜ (7)   KRCO ⬜⬜⬜⬜ (17)

EECUNMNGORTAE ⬜⬜⬜⬜⬜⬜⬜⬜⬜⬜⬜⬜⬜ (22, 14, 20)   SAMGESA ⬜⬜⬜⬜⬜⬜⬜ (5, 12)

⬜⬜⬜⬜⬜ , ⬜⬜⬜⬜⬜⬜⬜ , ⬜⬜⬜⬜⬜⬜⬜
1 2 3 4 5   6 7 8 9 10 11 12   13 14 15 16 17 18 19 20 21 22

Word Find:

Find and circle the ten words or phrases that may signal the onset of labor.

```
T O X V S C O N T R A C T I O N S H O
L B U Q R O A K L S N R W K L A E M T
J I K M U C U S P L U G D G Q U W R F
V O G U V F T L U X D M P O I S R L C
K C O H S W C R H V K Y E J O E N X R
N R U P T U R E O F M E M B R A N E S
D A J Z Q E V L F E Y B A C K A C H E
A M W F C K N P M S N E Q N V D O X R
G P A K D B D I A R R H E A Z W R K M
I S P S T O W Z N E S T I N G R I S W
P D U F N U M P I G T O J V D F H I L
```

Labor and Birth Questionnaire

Mail this questionnaire to your childbirth educator as soon as possible after birth

Your name _____

Partner's name _____

Baby's birthdate _____

Baby's name _____

Weight _____ Length _____ Sex _____

Number of children prior to this birth _____

Doctor/midwife present at the birth_____

Hospital/Birth Center _____

Dates of classes attended _____

Childbirth educator _____

Number of classes mother attended _____

Number of classes partner attended _____

How much time did you practice each week? _____

Picture of new baby or new family

Labor and Birth Experience

Type of birth: Vaginal _____   Cesarean birth _____

Was this a normal, full-term, uncomplicated pregnancy?   Yes _____   No _____   If not, please explain _____
_____

Was labor induced?   No _____   Yes _____   If yes, how?   Medication to soften /ripen cervix _____ ;   Pitocin _____ ;
by healthcare provider rupturing membranes _____ .

If labor was induced, what was the reason given for the induction? _____

How did you know that labor had begun? _____

If the birth was by cesarean, when were you told that a cesarean would have to be done? _____

What was the reason given for the cesarean? _____
_____

During labor, did the doctor rupture your membranes?   No _____   Yes _____

If yes, at approximately how many centimeters dilation? _____

Prior to birth, what was your rating on the "Pain Medications Preference Scale" (page 98)? _____

(continued on back)

How long did you labor at home? _____

What was the approximate length of labor? _____ Time spent pushing? _____

How many hours were you in the hospital before birth? _____

What medications were given during labor? _____

What medications were given during pushing? _____

How did you feel about these medications? _____

_____

Location of birth: Birthing room (LDR, LDRP) _____   Delivery room _____

Describe how you pushed. _____

Did you have an episiotomy? _____   Any tears of perineum? _____

Were forceps or a vacuum extractor used? _____   If yes, what was the reason? _____

Who was with you during labor? _____

Who was with you during the birth? _____

Describe briefly the type of guidance and support that you received from:

   Doctor/Midwife _____

   _____

   Nursing staff _____

   _____

   Labor partner _____

What were the positive aspects of your birth experience? _____

_____

What were the negative aspects of your birth experience? _____

_____

Were you able to keep your baby with you immediately after birth? _____ If yes, for how long? _____

Describe your feelings at that time. _____

Did you have rooming-in? _____

If rooming-in was not available, were you able to get your baby for frequent feedings? _____

How are you feeding your baby?   Breast _____   Formula _____

If the baby is a boy, did you have him circumcised?   No _____   Yes _____

Now that you have had a chance to use your knowledge, do you think any areas should have been stressed in greater detail? Include comments on class, class content, and/or instructor. _____

_____

If you could change any aspect of your birth experience, what would it be? _____

_____

What advice or recommendations do you have for couples delivering at this hospital/birth center? _____

_____

Mother's Labor and Birth Summary

	What were you feeling? (physically and emotionally)	What helped you the most to cope?	What did partner do that was helpful?	Comments or suggestions
Early Labor				
Active Labor				
Transition				
Pushing				
Postpartum				

May I share this questionnaire with future classes?   Yes _____   No _____

Labor Partner's Birth Report

Initially, how did you feel about taking the classes with your partner? _____

_____

_____

_____

Did your concerns about childbirth change as a result of the classes? _____

_____

_____

_____

As a labor partner, were you adequately prepared to help your partner? _____

_____

_____

_____

What should have been covered more thoroughly in class? _____

_____

_____

_____

How often did you practice with your partner outside of class? _____

_____

_____

_____

What specific problems did your partner have during labor, and what did you do to help? _____

_____

_____

_____

Was her labor what you expected? _____

_____

_____

_____

Were you with your partner during birth? _____ How did you feel? _____

_____

_____

What suggestions would you give to other prospective labor partners? _____

_____

_____

Add any additional comments regarding course content, instructor, or hospital/birth center experience. _____

_____

_____